NATURAL THERAPY

Good Health Through Natural Therapy

EK Ledermann MD, FFHom, MRCPsych

Kogan Page

First published 1976
by Kogan Page Limited,
116a Pentonville Road, London N1 9JN

ISBN 0 85038 141 X

Printed by A. Wheaton & Co, Exeter

Dedicated to my mother

Contents

Introduction 1

1 The rising tide of illness 3
The role of conventional medicine; increasing illness: the facts;
some enemies of health – wrong food and harmful social habits;
dangers of smoking, alcohol, coffee and tea; the stress of life;
personal responsibility for health: an urgent need

2 The principles of natural therapy 17
Health and wholeness; natural stimulation; limitations of natural
therapy

3 Food and your health 23
Science and your diet; nutritional imbalance; wholeness of the
soil; degraded and unnatural food; natural therapy and diet – the
various diets, including fasting, raw fruit and vegetable diet, full
diet, additions; psychodietetics of natural therapy: hunger,
appetite, custom, symbolization; conclusion

4 Health and your bowel 61
Food and its fibre content: the need for roughage; the bowel
flora; natural elimination

5 The breath of life 67
Air pollution and your lungs; breathing and rhythm

6 Natural stimulation and your skin 71
Skin: not just a body envelope; surface elimination; heat treatment; cold treatment; Father Kneipp's water cure; combinations
in hydrotherapy; air treatment; sun treatment

7 Posture, exercise and relaxation 86
Your spine; standing, sitting and walking; a system of exercises; aerobics; autogenic training

8 Allies to Natural Therapy 107
Homoeopathy; acupuncture; osteopathy; chiropractic; massage

9 Twelve case histories 120
Recurrent boils; ulcerative colitis and virus infection of skin; osteo-arthritis; varicose ulcers; cirrhosis of the liver; catarrhal child; rheumatoid arthritis; heart failure; advanced nephritis; acne vulgaris; multiple sclerosis; acute sinusitis

Notes 135

Index 143

Introduction

Are you one of the many people who are becoming worried about our unnatural and damaging 20th century life style? If so, this book is intended to give you support and guidance. It embodies my experience as a doctor in private and hospital practice for over forty years, during which time I have treated patients suffering from both physical and mental illnesses.

My interest in Natural Therapy began when I was a young doctor in Germany, and over the years I have become convinced that civilized people become ill largely as the result of their increasingly unnatural way of life. Too many of us seek relief through the prescription of drugs for every mental and physical ailment. But we still possess, and can call upon, innate natural resources for good health. These resources must be fully mobilized to prevent illness and to effect recovery.

The central concept of Natural Therapy is that of *wholeness*. The Natural Therapist recognizes that illness is often the result of wrong, unnatural living which has affected the whole person. So Natural Therapy relies on changing the everyday attitudes and habits of the patient – modifying diet in accordance with sound natural principles, prescribing exercises, and setting up a series of natural stimuli to which the patient's innate vitality should respond. Natural Therapy urges people to respect the needs of their minds and bodies, and to act accordingly, both in health and in sickness. Natural Therapy also aims to help people by showing them that they need not rely on drugs and tobacco, and on 'social' stimulants like coffee, tea and alcohol, but can use their intelligence and accept responsibility for their own well-being.

Food is a very important factor in healthy living. Natural

Therapy recognizes the harm that results from the unnecessary impoverishment and degradation of food – which is the contribution to modern civilization by the food-growing and processing industries. The Natural Therapist expects to give guidance about the amounts and proportions of the various foods that are needed for the body and mind to function healthily. At the same time, he has to realize that we must live in society as we find it and that eating habits are, to some extent, a response to the stresses and strains that society imposes on us (and not merely a response to intensive advertising campaigns by food and drink manufacturers). So his approach is sensible and tolerant – Natural Therapy allows for the need of individual variations in diet, as in the other forms of treatment. While recognition of the significance of food is basic to Natural Therapy and to its conception of bodily wholeness, a Natural Therapist treats *all* the main functions of the patient's body. An improvement in any of these functions is not only of benefit to the particular organ immediately concerned but also to the *whole person*. Attention to breathing, to the skin, to posture, to relaxation, to exercise and to the bowels – each is of the greatest importance.

Natural Therapy works more effectively when certain auxiliary forms of treatment are added. In later chapters, this book outlines how homoeopathic medicine enhances the response to stimuli administered by the Natural Therapist. Manipulation (especially of the spine), and massage give patients further help in recovering from the strains of living, and acupuncture is a means of restoring a healthy equilibrium to the various disturbed functions. Ranging over matters which are of vital importance to health, this book introduces Natural Therapy to all those in search of a healthier, saner, happier life.

1 The rising tide of illness

Our subject is health as understood by the Natural Therapist.
The conventional doctor is also concerned with the health of his
patient and is relied upon to relieve or cure both physical and
mental ailments.

So what are the differences in approach between the conventional doctor and the Natural Therapist? Why should we question
the methods of modern medical science? With its vast army of
dedicated and highly trained practitioners, supported by the full
weight of research being carried out all over the world, medicine
occupies an exalted position in civilized society. To challenge its
unique claim to authority, we must first examine the nature of
conventional medical science, and then evaluate its successes and
its failures.

The role of conventional medicine

Conventional medical science, like any other science, works by a
process of *analysis*, a process which deals with problems by
isolating them. Although doctors are aware of the patient's total
personality, recognizing the unity of body and mind in psychosomatic illness, their training leads them to *fragmentation*, to the
search for specific causes and their effects. They are concerned
with *parts* of the body or the mind rather than with the whole
person.

This analytical approach has yielded valuable results. For
instance, in the field of mental illness, many patients gain a
measure of relief from their anxiety and other emotional troubles
through being prescribed drugs which act on the brain. In the
case of depression, electric convulsions are also used.

In the realm of physical diseases, the achievements are even higher. After a particular disease has been isolated in the diagnosis, it is frequently successfully treated by the specific remedy – infectious diseases are cured with antibiotics and others prevented, or made milder, by immunization; heart failure is helped by digitalis; diabetes by insulin; pernicious anaemia by vitamin B12. The hyperactivity of the thyroid gland is reduced by an appropriate drug, sluggish kidneys are stimulated by another, skin irritation is relieved by certain ointments. The analytical approach has also enabled surgeons to perform brilliant operations, removing diseased parts, such as inflamed appendices, gall bladders and cancerous growths. These are just a few examples of the ways in which doctors help their patients.

Not only do individual patients benefit from the applications of medical science, whole populations are saved from serious epidemics through the activities of public health authorities, which ensure pure water and clean milk and are concerned with hygiene in general.

Increasing illness: the facts

While the applications of medical research to conventional medicine will undoubtedly lead to many further successes, the overall amount of ill-health shows no sign at all of diminishing, In fact, all the available figures indicate an *increase* in disease in the population at large. Although modern medicine has developed treatments for a large range of illnesses, both trivial and serious, man on the whole does not seem to be getting healthier. Tuberculosis is no longer the scourge it used to be, but deaths from lung cancer and coronary thrombosis are increasing alarmingly. Such serious ailments are caused primarily by the mode of living of modern 'civilized' man. They are largely avoidable. This is a central argument of the Natural Therapist. Insisting that the *whole* person must be treated, he encourages us to change our life-style to one that makes, for instance, lung cancer (through smoking) and heart trouble (through smoking, unhealthy diet, excessive stress and too little exercise) much less likely.

It is necessary for us now to look at a few facts and figures in order to understand the scale of the problem facing medicine today.

The facts concerning illness in the modern world are truly alarming. Not the least disturbing aspect is the growth in *iatrogenic* disease – disease actually created by the medical profession! The growing demands of the sick are most often met by the prescription of an increasing range of drugs which are potentially harmful. And this is not only true for the terrible, exceptional, example of the thalidomide tragedy.

It is estimated by one authority that 'from 10 per cent to 15 per cent of patients in our general hospitals are suffering to a greater or lesser extent from our effects to treat them – from what have optimistically been called diseases due to medical progress'! This author does not blame individual doctors for this sad state of affairs; he does not call for greater care in prescribing. The fault lies not in negligence but in the very essence of scientific medicine, as a result of which the balance of nature has been upset. 'Our powers over nature in applied pharmacology have extended so far that nature seems to have become retaliatory and is exacting a heavy retribution.[1] 'It has been recorded from a large hospital in the USA that 5 per cent of in-patients suffered *major* toxic reactions consequent to diagnostic or therapeutic measures before or after admission, and it was concluded that iatrogenic disease could be regarded as one of the commonest conditions encountered during the survey.' This serious indictment has been confirmed.[2] Side-effects from drugs play an important part in causing ill-health.

None of this need surprise us when we consider that, in Britain alone, more than 10,000 million tablets of the aspirin, phenacitin or paracetamol type are consumed each year, and that 250,000 people are taking five or more analgesics daily.[3]

Apart from drug-induced illness, the extent of ill-health in our communities is quite staggering. An English survey in 1971 revealed that 95 per cent of those questioned had experienced some symptoms of ill-health in the previous two weeks. In a British national survey, nine-tenths of the adults interviewed reported symptoms from the previous two weeks – an average of

3·9 symptoms per person.[4] A further indication of the failure of modern medicine is given by examining the *increase* in reported illness over recent years, in spite of increasing medication. In the USA in 1960, restricted activities due to illness or injury amounted to 2,830,000 days, in 1972 to 3,402,000 days.[5] Another investigation covered four countries: Great Britain, West Germany, Italy and Czechoslovakia, and the years 1966 to 1967 compared with the years 1950 to 1951, showed a rise of 34 per cent in absence from work owing to ill-health.[6]

In Great Britain, the number of new claims (sickness benefit, etc) for sickness and invalidity in 1973 was ten million, an increase of about 250,000 (2·6 per cent) over 1972.[7] The expense of the British drug bill is colossal. Some drugs are bought without prescription. They cost £100,000,000 a year, to which the sum of £300,000,000 must be added to cover prescribed drugs.[8] But this is only a fraction of the American cost.

Mental illness claims a large share. The figures reveal that in the USA in 1955 the estimated number of in- and out-patients suffering from a psychiatric disorder was 1,675,000, but that this figure rose to 4,038,000 in 1971.[9]

One writer describes the present situation in Britain in these terms: 'There must be few people in our society who are without first-hand experience of mental disorder. At some time most have had to endure the strain and tribulation of schizophrenia, depressive illness or a suicidal act involving a member of the family. . . . In Britain, one woman in six and one man in nine is treated for a psychiatric disorder in hospital during some stage in the lifespan.'[10]

If one considers the figures for physical illnesses, a few examples reflect the situation. It is calculated that three per cent of women in Britain suffer from rheumatoid arthritis. The upward trend in death from heart disease is even more disturbing. In America, the deaths per 100,000 population from ischaemic heart disease and related diseases of the heart amounted to 285·4 in 1950, but increased to 328 in 1972. The actual number of deaths from these conditions were 666,665 in 1970 and 683,100 in 1972. Deaths from the various forms of cancer also rose alarmingly:

139·8 deaths per 100,000 population in 1970; in 1972, 166·6 with the total number of deaths 346,930.[11] In the United States, a rise of one per cent in the death rate had been noted during recent years, but the figures for 1975 reveal an increase of *five* per cent, five times the anticipated frequency! An explanation for this frightening 'cancer boom' is now sought by the Center for Health Statistics. Hormones, prescribed for women during the change of life, pollution of the atmosphere and of food are under suspicion.[12]

Let us now look at some of the underlying reasons for this depressing picture.

Some enemies of health: wrong food and harmful social habits
There seems little doubt that much illness is caused by the consumption of unhealthy food. This fact is demonstrated by the statistics on dental caries where it is the small minority that has no tooth decay. In a British survey, fewer than three young people (aged between 16 and 31 years) in 1,000, or 0·3 per cent were found to have 28 or more sound teeth.[13] It is not only the amount of tooth decay that is so alarming; the figures for dental illness are indicative of an overall state of bad health in the population.

As Dr Macpherson Lawrie says in his *Nature Hits Back*: 'And do we suppose, for a moment, that the cause which ruins teeth confines its attack to one department? It attacks general development, and this impairment in development is demonstrated very forcibly by the standard of "womanhood" and "manhood" which emerges from the early city train. The cause which ruins teeth does more than ruin teeth. It attacks our vigour, our glands, our mental qualities of health, and our sexual development and function. Today, throughout our land, nerves which instantly lose their poise if strained, depressions, and sexual abnormalities abound. Today . . . the symptoms of glandular disease are rampant . . .'

Dr Lawrie considers that incorrect nutrition is the cause of this deterioration in health. His answer to why this explanation has not been universally recognized is as follows: 'Incorrect nutrition today is unchallenged as a cause, simply because corrective drugs have blinded and hypnotized the nation. The sale and consumption of corrective drugs is seldom attacked, yet they contribute very largely to disease. Corrective drugs relieve the early signs and symptoms of incorrect nutrition. They relieve constipation; they relieve the discomfort of dyspepsia; they soothe the frayed and stimulate the apathetic nerves. Corrective drugs enable incorrect nutrition to flourish. Pills and purgatives, digestive remedies, nerve sedatives and tonics permit the cause of constipation, of dyspepsia and 'nerves' to prosper, and it is *this cause*, persisting as it does in spite of them, which creates the later and more serious and permanent disorder.'[14]

Another scientist, Weston A. Price, a member of the Research Commission of the American Dental Association, and of the American Association of Physical Anthropologists, confirms that unnatural food ruins both teeth and general health. In his book, *Nutrition and Physical Degeneration – A Comparison of Primitive and Modern Diets and their Effects*, he shows how races all over the world lost their splendid teeth and physique when they began to consume refined foods in place of natural and unadulterated food.[15]

As Dr Macpherson Lawrie has pointed out, digestive upsets are a frequent complaint. W. G. Scott-Harden states: 'In Britain one in every hundred of the population requires investigation each year for symptoms relating to the upper digestive tract.'[16] Many of these sufferers have ulcers in the stomach or duodenum; others have cancer of the stomach. A further proportion do not show any organic lesion, but feel unwell and are unable to enjoy their food.

We shall be considering diet in detail in a later chapter. We should note at this stage that unbalanced meals are often taken in response to the stresses of modern life, and that we are all subjected to continuous campaigns to eat processed food that is harmful to health. But unhealthy eating is only one of the factors responsible for increasing illness in civilized man. We shall now consider some other damaging habits, starting with smoking.

Dangers of Smoking
Cigarette smoking increases the risk of developing ischaemic heart disease several fold. Cigarette smoking is also an important

cause of lung cancer. In 1963 well over 30,000 people in Britain died of lung cancer; most of them men and half of them under the age of sixty-five. In other words, many of these were premature deaths of people in their prime, during their working years, and there is little doubt that a good 90 per cent of them died because they smoked cigarettes.

There is a clear and a quantitative relationship between cigarette smoking and lung cancer. Smoking is now estimated to cause 100,000 deaths in Great Britain every year. In 1969, it was held responsible for the greater part of 38·6 million days of absence from work attributed to bronchitis.[17] In the United States of America, the total increase in the death rate, associated with cigarette smoking has been estimated, in men, to be a 70 per cent increase, less in women.

While the death rate from heart disease seems to be declining in the USA lately, the sharpest increase was recorded in chronic respiratory disease, bronchitis, emphysema and asthma. Smoking is largely responsible for chronic bronchitis which is often accompanied by emphysema and also aggravates asthma. These three ailments 'doubled between 1954 and 1960' in the USA.[18]

Smoking has been indicted as the 'biggest single avoidable menace to health in contemporary life in Britain'. It causes 'all told, ten times as many deaths as all cancers unrelated to smoking, put together'. A cigarette smoker's chances of dying in middle age are twice those of a non-smoker. This situation is brought home by the statistics: two out of every five heavy cigarette smokers are likely to die before the age of 65, compared with only one out of every five non-smokers.[19]

Smoking also harms the children of smokers. They are sick more frequently than the children of non-smokers, respiratory illness being again the most common trouble; the presence of tobacco smoke in the home has been blamed.[20] The unborn baby is adversely affected in the womb by the mother's smoking.

Alcohol

Those addicted to smoking damage their health, but they remain acceptable members of the community. In the case of alcohol, there is not only damage to health, but also the danger of losing self-respect and the respect of others.

In the USA, the number of alcoholics has been estimated at five million, and the disease has been listed as the fourth worst for shortening life.[21] In the final stage of his disease, the alcoholic becomes demented, has slurred speech, suffers from epileptic fits, and may also be subject to delusions and hallucinations.

The extent of alcoholism in Britain can be judged from the following extract from an article in *World Medicine* by John Camp: 'Britain is well on the way to having a million alcoholics by 1980, according to a report recently published by the Merseyside Council on Alcoholism. At the moment, says the report, about 700,000 addicts exist, of whom at least half are in a stage advanced enough to require immediate medical or psychiatric treatment'.[22] The number of women alcoholics is increasing, as they are, also, in America. They are more difficult to treat than men, as they have greater difficulties in readjusting their lives to sobriety.[23]

Drink in excess presents many insidious dangers to health, even to those who are not addicted to it. It reduces inhibition, which means that people behave without the usual restraint. They lose finer grades of judgement, the capacity to reflect and observe, and they also lose control over their emotions. Physical and mental efficiency are dangerously reduced when, for instance, someone who has been drinking, drives a car. Alcohol also affects the heart, damaging the heart muscle. There is loss of body heat through dilation of blood vessels, loss of appetite due to irritation of the lining of the stomach, often resulting in nutritional deficiencies. Furthermore, alcohol has a toxic effect on the liver, which leads to hepatic cirrhosis, and on the nerves, which leads to neuritis.

Coffee and tea
While the harmful effects of alcohol and smoking are well-known, there is widespread ignorance regarding the effects of ordinary tea and coffee, – effects which vary according to personal sensitivity. Many healthy people appear to take these beverages

without coming to harm, but the dangers from these stimulants must be pointed out and people whose health has broken down should replace them by harmless drinks, such as herb teas, dandelion coffee or fruit juices.

The book, *Coffee and Caffeine* by Dr Rolf Ulrich, gives a full account of the subject. As tea contains caffeine, the pharmacologically active ingredient in coffee, his findings apply to both tea and coffee. The author describes the absorption of caffeine from the intestinal tract. This varies greatly in different people. Even after ten to eleven hours, caffeine is still found in the urine, where it is excreted, and the effects on various organs are cited.

Caffeine causes a contraction of the heart and a rise in blood pressure due to spasm of small arteries. Dr Ulrich therefore voices the following warnings:

1 In arteriosclerosis (hardening of arteries, a common condition), the vascular effects of caffeine are longer lasting and stronger than in the case of a normal circulation

2 Caffeine represents a considerable additional burden on an arteriosclerotic vascular system

3 The rise in basal metabolism (the building up of the body from nutrients and the breaking down of tissue constituents into simpler substances) must be considered as part of this additional burden. The author concludes from these findings that patients who suffer from raised blood pressure should not consume any drinks containing caffeine.

The effect of caffeine on the blood vessels of the skin has been studied. They dilate, and thus in inflammatory skin diseases such as eczema or dermatitis the condition is aggravated by caffeine, which also increases itching. Because caffeine affects the blood vessels which supply the eye, there is danger from caffeine in cases of glaucoma, a condition in which the pressure within the eye is increased, frequently leading to blindness. Caffeine also stimulates the brain, evident in a speeding up of mental processes, but this is followed by a deterioration of mental performance, and people tend to be more fatigued after the initial boost. Sleeplessness after drinking tea or coffee occurs in sensitive people, especially those in whom the thyroid gland is over-active.

By hastening the circulation in the kidneys, caffeine increases the flow of urine, which is harmful to those who suffer from irritation of the bladder (this includes men with the common complaint of prostatic enlargement).

Caffeine increases further the secretion from the glands lining the stomach, stimulating the secretion of gastric juice. It thus aggravates stomach complaints, especially ulceration. After consuming coffee and tea, there is a temporary increase in muscular tone and in muscular output, but then fatigue and premature tiredness set in.[24]

While tea and coffee contain the same potentially harmful substance, there are important differences between them. There is first a difference in the quantity of caffeine in a cup of coffee and a cup of tea: brewed coffee contains 100–150 mg of caffeine per cup, tea only 60–75 mg. Instant coffee contains 86–99 mg and decaffeinated coffee only 2–4 mg. Cola drinks contain 40–60 mg per glass. Pharmacologists regard an intake of over 250 mg per day as large and, even for the person who is not particularly sensitive to caffeine, as harmful. This amount is often greatly exceeded, and people are not aware of the risk they are taking.

Because coffee is so much stronger than tea, coffee poisoning is far more likely to occur than tea poisoning. The nervous system is affected: the patient is irritable, unable to work and becomes very anxious. The skin becomes over-sensitive, and sleep is broken. When he (more often she) stops taking the coffee, withdrawal symptoms set in: more irritability, more nervousness, lethargy and again inability to work. There is also a withdrawal headache. These symptoms are temporarily relieved by drinking more coffee, which of course leads to a vicious circle. Apart from the nervous system, the heart and the blood vessels are over-stimulated and the digestive organs suffer: people complain of nausea, vomiting and diarrhoea when poisoned by caffeine. These severe symptoms do not as a rule occur after taking even fairly large quantities of tea.[25]

Coffee has been found to increase a person's risk of developing the feared heart attack (myocardial infarction). In one study it was discovered that those who drink more than five cups of coffee per day 'have about twice as great a risk of having an acute myocardial infarction as people drinking no coffee at all'.[26] As this risk does not occur in tea drinkers, one author assumes that the coffee bean is responsible, as it contains substances which cause blood clotting, a feature in the infarction, whereas tea does not contain such substances.[27] Coffee is also more likely to precipitate attacks of migraine than tea and can also, in the case of people who are sensitive to caffeine, cause gall bladder pain which is not found in tea drinkers.

In a recent article, published in the British Medical Journal attention has been drawn to the evidence, collected from a number of sources, that coffee drinking increases the risk of cancer in the bladder and in the kidneys.[28]

Tea is not only detrimental to health on account of its caffeine content. It contains other harmful chemical substances, called tannins. These have been made responsible for the inhibition of iron absorption from some foods, especially from vegetables. As iron is an essential element in the blood, a deficiency of iron, caused by tea drinking, leads to anaemia.[29]

The stress of life

Moderate drinking of tea and of coffee is clearly an acceptable social habit for healthy people, but the taking of excessive cups is something different: it is an ineffective method, used by the neurotic, to cope with the stresses of life. The extent of neurosis has been revealed by A. Ryle in his book *Neurosis in the Ordinary Family*. He found that 'Some 30 per cent or so of the population ... present with chronic or recurrent symptoms of emotional stress and tension. These are the more or less insecure, immature people with only partially-met dependent needs, whose adjustment to life is maintained only at the price of some restriction and of some symptoms'.[30] Apart from drinking many cups of tea and coffee and often smoking countless cigarettes, neurotics swallow vast quantities of tranquillizers and sedatives.

According to a recent article in the *British Medical Journal*, 'The annual number of prescriptions for tranquillizers and sedatives increased by 60 per cent in England and Wales between 1965 and 1970 until in that year 17·2 million prescriptions for these drugs were dispensed under the N(ational) H(ealth) S(ervice). (This figure does not take into account drugs prescribed in psychiatric institutions). There is evidence to suggest that the number is still increasing.'[31]

Stress is responsible for psychosomatic illnesses, for disturbances in the functions of the heart, lungs, stomach, bowels, muscles, and the nervous system. Many skin complaints are explicable on this basis. A disturbed function can lead to changes in structure. Ulcers in the stomach and duodenum, already mentioned as a frequent cause of ill-health, are partially caused by stress.

Ischaemic heart disease, discussed earlier, is aggravated by stress. The stressful situation which can lead to death from heart trouble may be the news of the death of a beloved person – or the anniversary of such an event. It may be caused by a loss of self-esteem, or even the excitement of joyous circumstances. The emotional stress causes changes in the brain and in the nervous system which, in turn, affect the action of the heart. A psychiatrist, Joseph Connolly, examined the significance of various emotional factors in the disease of the blood vessels of the heart. He found that frustration was important. It plays a part in work situations and in a person's social life. A person who suffers from what has been called 'status incongruity' is particularly at risk. He finds that his level of education does not match his occupation or the type of house in which he lives. He cannot form good relations with his neighbours, as his self-image prevents him from accepting the social life in his district. Such people show intense sustained drive, are eager to compete, very alert, engaged in many and diverse activities. They move fast, have explosive intonation in their speech, clench their hands and teeth, make unconscious gestures, are impatient and suffer from 'a chronic state of urgency'. (They are also apt to over-eat and to smoke heavily.)[32]

If people live in a community which strongly supports them, they are largely protected from the risk of stress diseases. Unfortunately human support is weakening in our society.

Children suffer particularly from the breaking up of their parents' marriage. Alvin Toffler has given us an account of the sources of stress in American society which is also valid, to a lesser or greater degree, for other Western communities. In his *Future Shock* he characterizes modern man as a restless person, always on the move towards a new place of work, towards a new job – which means towards new work associates and new social contacts. Under such conditions, his family becomes 'fractured', marriages are temporary, everything is transient.[33] This rootlessness must be considered an intolerable strain.

While we cannot hope to eliminate all the strains and stresses of our technological, competitive age, we can and must change our attitude if we are to achieve a better level of health. This fundamental reorientation will now be discussed.

Personal responsibility for health: an urgent need

What is the common attitude of the sick population? Brought up in the era of scientific medicine, they have been led to believe that their health is a matter solely for the trained doctor to understand. They have not studied the intricacies of mind and body and therefore do not accept responsibility for their own health. Misled by their doctors, their orientation is towards disease.

There is widespread faith in the pills and mixtures which scientific medicine has created, and the idea seems to be that the more medicine you swallow, the better you will feel. People look for quick relief of any discomfort, and such relief is given by the products of the drug industry. Clever advertisements promise strength and better health. Patients are lured into buying medicines at the chemist's shop, or asking their doctors for various prescriptions after having seen pictures of people who show radiant 'health' as the result of some wonder 'cure'. There is no mention of the fact that the effects are purely palliative – and that, often, such preparations cause serious damage to health, as we have seen.

People take pills for indigestion and constipation, rather than regulating their diet, which would make such medication unnecessary. They reject the need for discipline. They know that over-eating, especially of sugar, makes them fat. So they ask their doctors for medicines which will artificially reduce their appetite. They are not prepared to accept the feeling of hunger which is necessary if they are to lose superfluous fat. If people do not fall asleep immediately on going to bed, they ask for sleeping tablets which induce sleep but also a 'hangover' the next day. If they are emotionally upset, they expect to be calmed by taking sedatives, instead of facing the disturbance which is upsetting them and trying to deal with it. The medical profession is to blame for failing to encourage patients to take responsibility for their own health. Doctors treat people as objects of science and not as free persons. By prescribing appetite suppressant drugs for the greedy, and cough mixtures for the smoker, the doctor promotes irresponsibility. Also, if he himself leads an unhealthy life, as is often the case, he sets a bad example to his patients and thus encourages them to ignore the rules of health. (Acting irresponsibly in regard to his own health, he also does so in regard to that of his patients.)

Doctors' and patients' attitudes towards health (usually unconsciously held) stem from the scientific-analytic approach which, as we have seen, is also responsible for the suffering caused by iatrogenic illness. A different attitude which does not produce these harmful consequences will now be outlined.

2 The principles of natural therapy

We have seen how and why the fragmented approach of modern analytical medicine fails to do justice to health. With the ever-increasing specialization that is taking place in medicine, the doctor himself is liable to lose sight of the whole person. Since the general practitioner is trained by specialists at medical school, his conception of medicine is based on the subdivision of the patient's body and mind – at the expense of wholeness.[1]

Health and wholeness

In contrast to conventional medicine, Natural Therapy is founded on the idea of *wholeness*, a wholeness which stands for health and harmony. Even if this cannot always be maintained under the stressful conditions of modern life, the principle of wholeness remains fundamental. After any disturbance – whether a feverish illness or an emotional upset – has shaken the whole person, a return to equilibrium, to wholeness, constitutes recovery. The whole is more than the agglomeration of parts; they are bound together by the whole, they function under its auspices.

The idea of wholeness is basic in the study of living organisms. The science of physiology illustrates its significance. The heart is known as the organ that supplies the whole body with blood, the kidneys are understood as the organs which eliminate certain waste products for the benefit of the whole body. Each individual organ is viewed in its relation to the whole body. The centres (situated in the central nervous system) which regulate tempera-ture, and breathing and other vital functions play a crucial role in preserving wholeness. In fact, maintenance of wholeness is the

very feature which distinguishes the living organism from non-
living things, and all Natural Therapy treatment relies on nature's
power to preserve or restore the wholeness which equals health.

By making wholeness its central concept, Natural Therapy pays
attention to the vital factors on which health (wholeness) depends.
To the Natural Therapist, illness is likely to be the result of wrong
living which has affected the whole person, even though the
trouble may manifest itself only in one or several parts. Wrong
feeding, eating food which has been produced wrongly, neglect
of exercise, failure to pay attention to the skin and the bowels,
ignorance of how to breathe properly, lack of sleep and of
relaxation, poor posture – all these are understood to be causes of
illness. Although ideal natural wholesome conditions cannot be
established under the unnatural circumstances of our civilization,
it is possible to help a patient or to prevent illness by modifying
the strain.

Achieving wholeness
The medical scientist, guided by the analytical-specific approach,
prescribes a diet only in the case of such diseases as obesity or
diabetes. The Natural Therapist, on the other hand, prescribes
a diet for every patient who is not eating in accordance with the
principles of wholeness (the definition of wholesome food is given
in Chapter 3). In the same way, breathing exercises are given not
only to people suffering from respiratory troubles, but are
considered in *all* cases, for correct breathing is one of the vital
functions affecting the whole person. Muscular exercises are not
prescribed just to strengthen weakened muscles, as is the practice
in analytical-specific medicine, but they are given to *all*, in order
to improve general health. Skin treatment is carried out through
the use of natural stimuli: water, sun and air and, once again,
such treatment is not confined to cases of skin disease but is
prescribed for *all* sick people: the skin is an important organ
which fulfils functions that are vital for the person as a whole.
The same considerations apply to the bowel, to posture, to rest
and to relaxation. By improving these vital functions, the Natural
Therapist not only improves general health but also provides help

to the particular part where the general disease shows itself (the
stomach, the liver, the skin, and so on). In his view the body
functions as a whole, and whatever is done to improve one part
will benefit all the others.

Natural Therapy basically consists in changing the conditions
of living, and this involves a change in habits. By eliminating
certain food from the diet, by applying cold water to the skin
(generally not used to cold water), by prescribing exercises for the
physically inactive, and by other measures which affect vital
functions, a *natural stimulus* is set up to which the patient's innate
vitality is expected to respond. Thus, Natural Therapy can be
defined as a method which employs natural stimuli to counter
the effects of unnatural, unhealthy living.

Natural stimulation

Natural stimuli are graded according to their intensity. Cold
water has a stronger effect than lukewarm water. Natural stimuli
applied to the skin can be varied by exposing a larger or smaller
area; for instance, a cold compress around the neck is less
effective than one which covers the whole body. With regard to
sunlight, the treatment is graded according to the size of the skin
area, the length of time it is exposed, and the intensity of the sun's
rays. So far as diet is concerned, the range extends from a fast on
water only; to raw juices, raw fruits and raw vegetables; to the
addition of dairy produce and of cooked vegetables, and finally
to a full mixed diet including meat and fish. Tea, coffee, refined
sugar and refined flour would not be included, as they are potentially harmful.

The natural stimulus is adjusted to the particular patient's
needs and ability to respond. The needs are dictated by the
seriousness of his or her condition; for instance, in a case of
congestion of the lungs, a fast and a whole-body compress may be
essential, whereas, in a case of bronchitis, a small compress
around the chest and a raw food diet may be sufficient. With
regard to the patient's response, the following factors are
considered:

1 *The constitution*: People differ considerably in their ability to

stand up to heat, to cold to fasting, and so on. For instance, take the constitution of the skin: its ability to respond to cold water can be judged by its degree of firmness and its readiness to perspire and, in responding to sunlight, people differ in their capacity to produce pigment.

2 *Previous habits*: In judging how a patient will respond to Natural Therapy, the Natural Therapist enquires into his individual history. Someone who has always washed in cold water can be expected to tolerate a large cold compress, but someone who has always indulged in hot baths may find intensive cold unbearable. The person who has lived on a food-reform diet may need a period on raw salads, while the one who has eaten a mixed diet, with tea, coffee and alcohol, may respond better to a lacto-vegetarian regime.

3 *Age*: Age is another factor which must be taken into account when deciding on the intensity of the natural stimulus. Babies cannot stand exposure to cold, nor deprivation of fluids. Very old people also need warmth; their resistance to a fast may be insufficient and they cannot be expected to stand up to a great deal of physical exercise. Between these extremes of age, all degrees of tolerance are met.

4 *The effects of diseases*: Chronic infections (such as tuberculosis or chronic bronchitis), degenerative diseases (such as arterio-sclerosis) and malignant disease (such as cancer) weaken vitality. In all such conditions, only a mild form of treatment is used.

5 *The Mind*: A change in the mode of living not only affects a patient's body but also his mind, and his mind must be ready for the change. He must be prepared to forgo certain foods and drinks in order to achieve better health. He must also be ready to accept social inconvenience, as his family and friends may not be sharing his new way of life. He therefore needs courage and determination, which will often earn him respect from others. He must not conceive of the new regime as a punishment, or a deprivation, but as an adventure which he will find of absorbing interest. He will gain encouragement from the fact that, by adopting a new mode of living, he will be improving his health. For above all, he must recognize his own responsibility for his state of health and must abandon the idea that it is up to the doctor to make him well.

Limitations of Natural Therapy

The Natural Therapist holds a central position, for his approach to health and disease is basic, and what he practices is *not* fringe medicine. He must, however, avoid dogmatism and fanaticism. No school of medicine can claim to be all-sufficient. While it is correct to trust the self-healing power of nature, it is not correct to trust this power absolutely. If a patient fails to respond to natural treatment, or if his condition is such that no response to natural treatment can be expected, then the resources of scientific modern medicine must be made available. (Other methods which will be discussed later, and which are auxiliary to Natural Therapy, can enlarge the scope of natural treatment, but limitations of even this combined approach still exist and must be faced.)

The Natural Therapist must assess his patient's condition and decide according to his interpretation of the symptoms when a change from Natural Therapy to conventional medical treatment is demanded. For instance, an attack of diarrhoea can be understood as an attempt, made by the body, to eliminate toxic material for the benefit of the whole organism. In this case, the patient will be put on a fast with sufficient water to replace the lost fluid. On the other hand, the diarrhoea may be due to some virulent infection, and may weaken the patient, and in this case the responsible Natural Therapist abandons the natural treatment and stops the diarrhoea by using an antibiotic. A fever may be regarded as a beneficial effort, on the part of nature, to burn up toxic matter; here a short fast will be called for and the patient will feel better when his temperature returns to normal. A fever may, however, be due to the invasion of the body by a dangerous germ, and may have to be stopped by a drug to prevent bodily resistance being overwhelmed and the patient succumbing.

Emergencies necessitating surgery must be recognized, and

immediately treated accordingly. A perforation of the stomach cannot be treated by natural methods, only by a life-saving operation. An attack of acute appendicitis can be treated with a fast, but the Natural Therapist takes a risk which may not be justified if surgical help is readily available.

Mental (emotional) illness presents a further limitation. It is true that living a life as far as possible in accordance with Nature (i.e. avoiding stimulants, drugs and other unwholesome interference) promotes mental as well as physical health. But adopting unhealthy habits, such as smoking, drinking and taking drugs that affect the mind, is often the manifestation of a disturbed mind which cannot be cured by the prescriptions of Natural Therapy. Natural treatment may in fact aggravate a mental disturbance if it promotes an abnormal mental attitude. For instance, an unbalanced mind might well become more unbalanced after a fast. A person obsessed by ideas of purity might become even more fanatic as a result of adopting measures which are aimed at elimination of toxins from the body. A girl, haunted by the fears of getting fat, might seize on a restricted diet and die of anorexia nervosa. Therefore, the Natural Therapist accepts the mental as well as the physical limitations of his methods – methods which rely on a favourable response from the patient's mind as well as from his body.

Having clarified the principles on which Natural Therapy is based, let us now see how they can be applied. Our first concern will be the relationship between food and health.

3 Food and your health

Science and your diet

Textbooks of dietetics deal with the various components which make up your diet. These are water, protein, carbohydrates, fats, vitamins, mineral salts and trace elements. Tables have been compiled giving the amounts of these items needed by men, women and children. Other tables provide information about the chemical energy derived from different types of food, measured in calories (a calorie being the amount of heat energy required to raise the temperature of 1,000 grammes of water by one degree centigrade).

The tables which dietitians use to assess food requirements show the calorific yield of different foods. This approach implies that such an analysis gives valid information about human nutrition. This claim has been refuted by Dr Hall, a biochemist working at McMaster University in Ontario. In his recent book *Food for Nought: The Decline in Nutrition* he calls for an entirely fresh scientific approach which is not just based on chemical analysis of food but which takes into account the complexities of the interactions occurring within the microscopic structures that compose our bodies. He has pointed out that the addition of chemicals (which will be discussed later in this chapter) may be harmless in isolation, but harmful in combination with each other. Hall insists that all the environmental agents which influence the consumer of food must be taken into account, and he includes social, political, economic and ethical factors.[1]

The follower of Natural Therapy, while agreeing with Dr Hall's criticism, does not wait until the 'new' science of nourishment has been created. He is guided by the idea of wholeness, and we shall see how this idea can lead to practical conclusions about correct nutrition without delay. Calculation is impossible, for the individual person is unique in his nutritional needs and varies in his own lifetime in response to biological, social and emotional forces. Even conventional dietetic science recognizes variations of calorific needs amounting to 20 per cent. Thus a man of a certain height and weight and a certain age, resting in bed, might need 2,200 calories per day, while an identical man, also resting but with a lower energy consumption, would balance his needs with an intake of 1,800 calories.

To the Natural Therapist, your body is not just a machine which needs fuel for its performance, and it is not sufficient to think in terms of calories or energy units. Two examples of imbalance – obesity and the saccharine disease – demonstrate the complexity of the nutritional problem.

Nutritional imbalance
Obesity
Obesity is a very common nutritional disorder of the affluent society. In America, one in five men and one in four women over the age of 20 weigh at least 20 pounds above their ideal weight. 50 per cent of London employees of the BP Company were overweight, according to a study by a life insurance company. In another survey, 13 per cent of 2,000 adults were found to be currently trying to lose weight and 25 per cent had tried to do so within the previous year. American life insurance investigations have proved that overweight people die younger.[2]

Obesity often starts in childhood and persists throughout life. It is apt to lead, in later years, to diseases of the blood vessels, the gall bladder and the heart. It also causes severe emotional distress, as the fat person suffers from being, and feeling, unattractive. The fat person battles against being fat. In the study of obese children it has been found that 'most children in Britain consume more calories and a greater amount of carbohydrate than they require, yet only a small proportion become grossly obese'.[3] Therefore, people differ in the way in which their bodies make use of food.

It has been claimed that obesity is inherited and that the fact that many members of the same family are fat cannot simply be explained on the grounds that they are all in the habit of eating too much. Fat stores may be more or less available for oxidation (burning-up) and for the depositing of fat or its constituents.

The analytical approach of scientific medicine has isolated a centre in the brain which regulates an individual's appetite. If this 'appestat' does not function properly, obesity may be the result.

The psychological factor must also be considered. For some people, food is 'the short-term panacea for all emotional stress'. These are people who suffer emotional strain and who 'have learned to turn to food whenever they become anxious or upset', they therefore 'seek solace in food very frequently'.[4] The type of food which provides this consolation, and at the same time produces obesity, is carbohydrate; that is, sugar and flour, eaten in the form of sweets, bread, cake, ice-cream, and so on.

Finally there are important social-cultural considerations. To be overweight is socially unacceptable among the richer people who, therefore, make efforts at slimming. It is, however, quite acceptable amongst the poorer people, the 'lower' social classes. Hence 'it is very unlikely that a plump middle-aged woman whose family say they prefer her like that, and who cannot believe that she is in any way at risk, will accept with any enthusiasm advice to lose weight.'[5]

Saccharine disease
What is the menacing-sounding 'saccharine disease'? This term has been developed to cover all these disorders of the body which are due to the widespread habit of consuming much too much refined carbohydrates. This habit really is a menace. People today eat staggering quantities of these substances, as the following figures show. In 150 years the amount of sugar we consume per head has jumped eightfold, from a reasonable 15lb in 1815 to 1965's figure of 123 lb. This is equivalent to a daily consumption of 5 oz (140 grammes) per person – the sugar obtained from some 2½ lb (1·130 kg) of sugar beet.[6] It has been pointedly asked: 'Who

would consume that quantity daily of the parent food?'

This change in eating habits has seriously upset the balance of the whole organism. It is now claimed that not only obesity – the all too obvious result of over-indulgence in sugar and flour – but a whole range of other conditions which plague modern man can be recognized as manifestations of the saccharine disease.

The connection between the consumption of refined carbohydrates and the loss of sound teeth has already been mentioned, but diabetes mellitus should also be looked at in relation to the over-consumption of carbohydrates. The pancreas (the gland which is mainly concerned with sugar metabolism) suffers when having to deal with an excess of carbohydrates, and studies in Natal support this contention. The Indians living there show a frequency of diabetes which is 'one of the highest in the world and probably ten times as high as in India itself – and their sugar consumption is nearly ten times as high too'.[7] It also maintained that saccharine disease has further manifestations: the refined diet causes unnatural loading of the colon which in turn leads to stasis and pressure on the venous return within the pelvis. Thus, varicose veins in the legs, enlargement of the veins within the scrotum and haemorrhoids are the result. Further proof is again provided by comparing people who live on unrefined foods with those who adopt the habit of food refinement. The two groups show significant differences with regard to the prevalence of ulcers in the stomach and in the duodenum. A connection has been made between these peptic ulcers and the over-consumption of refined carbohydrates: the refined carbohydrates enter the stomach without being accompanied by proteins (which have been eliminated through the refining process). The result is that the acid in the stomach is not neutralized, and this excess of acid contributes to the formation of ulcers.

But the range of saccharine disease extends further and includes coronary disease, in which the significance of tobacco smoking has already been stressed. High carbohydrate consumption has been strongly suggested as a further factor, for coronary disease and obesity are often associated, and diabetes and coronary disease also go hand in hand. Thus, as these two conditions are frequently caused by carbohydrate over-consumption, the inclusion of coronary disease in saccharine illness appears to be justified.

The various manifestations of saccharine disease confirm the Natural Therapist's conception that the organism functions as a whole, and that an imbalance in the diet has widespread harmful consequences for the whole person. Further confirmation can be found in the fact that over-eating of carbohydrates upsets the equilibrium of the bowel flora – the different types of micro-organisms which are present in the large bowel. This additional disturbance has been considered to be a contributory cause of inflammation of the appendix, the gall bladder and the kidney (pyelitis). All these conditions are common to Western man and, by contrast, are extremely rare in those communities which adhere to a diet which does not contain refined carbohydrates.[8]

Wholeness of the soil

The principles of biological wholeness include the wholeness of the soil. We have seen how the Natural Therapist conceives a person's health largely in nutritional terms and how he lays stress on wholesome food and on avoiding the many unwholesome things which people eat. However, food is only wholesome if it is grown in healthy soil. In the soil, as in the body of an animal or a human being, health is a matter of balance, and ill-health is equivalent with imbalance. In company with many organic gardeners, the Natural Therapist holds that modern agricultural techniques are responsible for imbalance within the soil and for a sickness of the land which, in turn, causes sickness in the animals which feed on the land and the human beings who derive their nourishment from the plants growing in the soil and from the animals.

As in conventional medicine, the 'scientific' approach in agriculture suffers from that short-sighted fragmentation which is characteristic of rigidly applied scientific method. As unhealthy soil is one where good crops cannot be raised, where plants suffer from diseases and where pests abound, to the Natural Therapist, these troubles are symptoms of disequilibrium. They call for organic farming, which means the use of humus. Humus is 'a product of the decomposition of animal and vegetable residues brought about through the agencies of micro-organisms. . . . It is organic matter, in the transition stage between one form of life and another. Once the inorganic passes into the organic, and this is a constant process, it is subject to continual change within the organic cycle, the variety in the forms of life through which it may pass being almost endless.'[9]

Humus is made by 'composting', for which there are different techniques. The heaped-up materials consist of mixed animal and vegetable wastes which include all vegetable and crop residues; furthermore, humus includes a base such as earth, wood ash, chalk, sea sand, or a mixture of these. The base reduces the acidity. In addition, the compost heap must contain air and water. In this collection of substances, intense fermentation sets in, which causes a rise of temperature, and the formation of a 'mycelium', composed of fungi. Now the material breaks up, with bacteria playing a leading part in the process. The Natural Therapist would agree with Sir Albert Howard that 'humus treatment confers on plants a power of disease resistance amounting in some cases almost to immunity, and that a like result is not, and cannot, be obtained by the use of artificial fertilizers.'[10]

The conventional 'scientific' method of dealing with plant disease consists in using sprays. DDT is effective, but the pests become resistant, just as some germs become resistant to antibiotics. The sprays are developed by the science of chemistry, but the science of chemistry, which deals with specific relationships between substances, is not capable of doing justice to the 'fountain of energy flowing through a circuit of soils, plants and animals, to soil fertility, the capacity of soil to receive, store and transmit energy.'[11] In conformity with his views on health and disease, the Natural Therapist believes that what is needed is research into the whole.[12]

The scientific agriculturalist may argue that he must aim at raising the yields of crops to feed as many people as possible and the organicist cannot deny the strength of this argument, for where soil is deficient, it is obvious that the deficiency should be

made good by artificial means. However, the introduction of
toxic chemical substances, used as pesticides, is not a replacement
of essential missing elements, as it represents dangerous interference with the life in the ⌐ ⁄il. Waste products of living things,
including their dead remains, are consumed by bacteria, enter
the life cycle and thus are never a risk. Artificial substances, on
the other hand, do not enter the life cycle and may accumulate in
the bodies of animals feeding from the soil. For instance, DDT
may be present in a plankton in a lake at the innocuous level of
0·04 per million, but it may be concentrated in a duck feeding
from the lake at a two thousand million times greater measure,
and may well be harmful to the person eating the duck. The
materials which farmers use to boost growth undergo conversion
in the soil, which results in the production of certain acids. In
this way, the alkali/acid balance is liable to be upset and, in turn,
plant growth may suffer. Recent medical research has pointed
to the danger to people which can arise from the acid end-
products of biological decomposition. A connection with the
formation of cancer has been suggested.[13]

The danger arising from one chemical fertilizer, nitrate, has
recently been revealed. Nitrate is used extensively, in the United
States at the rate of seven million tons per year, and the result
can be disastrous, as plants and animals are poisoned by this
substance if the soil structure is not well supplied with humus
and organic matter. Nitrates are converted into toxic nitrite.
When this is taken into the bodies of domestic animals, their
glands suffer and, in cows, the milk production diminishes. There
is a link with human cancer. The bodies of babies are particularly
sensitive to nitrite which enters the drinking water and may be
stored in spinach. Even a commercial preparation of spinach,
sold as baby-food, was found to contain a dangerous excess of
nitrite.[14] This example illustrates the risks which are taken when
the rate of plant growth is forced: such a risk must always be
kept in mind. Science offers the means of increasing yields; such a
policy may be justified by the need to feed more people, but after
the scientist has provided the technical means of interfering with
nature, he must check carefully on the possible side-effects. In

contrast, the Natural Therapist avoids these perils, since he refrains from interfering with natural growth.

Degraded and unnatural food

A Natural Therapist not only objects to the degradation of food as the result of interfering with the life in the soil; he also opposes other processes which deprive food of its natural qualities. Antibiotics promote the growth of cattle and, by giving these substances to their animals, farmers can greatly reduce the time it takes to bring them to market, but the antibiotic is also ingested by the person who eats the meat, and if he contracts a serious disease which needs to be treated with antibiotics, his own microbes may be found to be insensitive to the drug. The glands which produce hormones are also affected by a growth hormone, given to animals, which can cause widespread and unpredictable disturbances in people. It has been reported, for example, that this growth hormone is a 'recognized cancer producer', that 'an estimated 90 per cent of the cattle for the US market are fed this substance which can cause hormonal changes in humans', and that 'European Common Market countries have banned US beef' for this reason.[15]

Astonishing as it may seem, the contemporary convenience-food industry employs over fifteen hundred non-nutritive additives, many of which may have adverse effects on the people who consume them; for science cannot yet be expected to have discovered all the consequences of eating such superfluous 'cosmetic' ingredients. As Professor Shears points out, 'in the factories food is bleached, coloured, dehydrated, hydrolized, homogenized, emulsified, pasteurized, gassed, preserved chemically and canned', and he adds a warning with which the Natural Therapist would agree: 'Not only is there danger from toxic qualities of these processes but such toxicities are known to be destructive of vitamins.' There is a further danger to health from the treatment of drinking water with chlorine, aluminium sulphates, carbon, hydrated lime and fluoride.[16]

The processing of food destroys vitamins, but if, by way of compensation, vitamins are added later, the natural balance in

the food is still disturbed. Bread is a classic example. Vitamin B
is taken out of the flour in the manufacturing process. Synthetic
Vitamin B is added which, however, does not contain all the
natural ingredients which have been removed from the grain.
Vitamin E is lost. The enzymes, essential for proper assimilation,
are destroyed and cannot be replaced effectively.[17] Bread, a staple
diet for whole populations, has been effectively degraded for the
convenience of the food manufacturers, and we are persuaded to
prefer the degraded product.

Professor Shears insists that artificial flavouring 'has deceived
our flavour senses into taking foods not good for us'. He blames
these artificial agents for inducing a craving for those processed
carbohydrates.

Food preservation can add to the hazards. Nitrate, condemned
earlier as a fertilizer, is widely used for this purpose, particularly
in smoked fish and processed meats – for instance, in frankfurters,
luncheon meat, cured ham and cured beef. The risk of this
substance causing cancer, stressed before, has been confirmed by
a group of scientists in the USA.[18]

Losses of mineral salts and vitamins also occur during cooking,
which should therefore be confined to a minimum time. The
water in which vegetables have been cooked should be consumed
as it contains mineral salts. Exposure to light destroys vitamin
B2, hence storage in the dark and in the cold atmosphere of a
refrigerator is advisable. As important nutrients are deposited
under the skins of apples or potatoes, peeling them leads to
losses that should be avoided. The addition of salt lowers the
vitamin C content. With regard to cooking utensils, health-
conscious cooks should note that copper destroys vitamin C and
that aluminium combines with food to cause toxic effects in
susceptible people. Pyrex dishes, iron and steel are safe.

Well-prepared food will be a thing of the past if we are to
believe certain prophesies from advanced food technologists:
they envisage artificial foods. An article in *World Medicine* deals
with 'chemical' diets. It bears the misleading title: 'Making Food
Efficient', and states that 'completely chemically defined diets . . .
offer a high degree of chemical flexibility and are composed

solely of purified and discrete chemical constituents'. The authors claim that people can be maintained in good health on such a regime.[19]

This artificial diet may have a place in cases of special diseases where the particular abnormality can be dealt with in a specific manner, but a Natural Therapist cannot accept the plan to use an artificial chemical diet as a 'perfect biological replacement' for, to give one example, breast milk for babies. He would argue that breast milk contains numerous elements which nature has balanced and which not only nourish the baby but also provide immunity against infections. Cows' milk may not give the same protection, but it is also a natural product, whereas any chemical compound, however sophisticated, cannot be expected to match nature's equilibrium.

Milk contains protein, sugar, fat, salts and vitamins. This is nature's way of preparing food, and to isolate protein from other constituents may well upset the natural balance. The Natural Therapist therefore views with concern the efforts made by industry to synthesize proteins. Professor Jack Edelman recently discussed these products at a nutrition conference, mentioning meat substitutes and proteins derived from fungi and from yeast. These substances, when manufactured on a large scale, are more economic to produce than meat, and they are being tested on humans at present for 'palatability and long-term tolerance'.[20] Further details of the work of the food technologist are given in Professor Shears' book *Nutritional Science & Health Education.* People who believe in Natural Therapy would agree with Shears when he reminds us that 'the food technologists have foisted refined and sophisticated foods on the public [and] have con-tributed a good deal to the incidence of ill-health and what effect the proposed "food" may have is anybody's guess'. Shears reminds us of the evolution of man and of his eating habits: 'Our natural foods have evolved, as we have evolved, through cen-turies and a complete change to artificial [foods] might imperil the future – or mean no future at all!'[21]

J. G. Davis, past Chairman of the Society of the Chemical

Industry's Food Group, envisages the following startling situation for the year 2000: Economic synthesis of proteins, sugars, fats, carbohydrates, of all known vitamins and flavours.
Efficient extraction from leaves and waste vegetable matter and the making of protein by micro-organisms. All foods will be consumed from plastic packages and meals will be provided by vending machines. There will be a blend of the natural derivative (e.g. leaf protein) and the artificial synthesized product.[22] There is no natural wholeness in such foods.

Natural therapy and diet

Having established the principles on which the Natural Therapist bases his dietetic treatment, we must now look at some of the ways these principles are put into practice. It has already been explained that Natural Therapy involves the breaking of harmful habits and the evoking of responses by inducing the body to extract nourishment from a diet different from the faulty one on which it relied before. It is this difference which constitutes a natural stimulus. There are numerous ways of applying this principle, and one of them is the following, rather drastic, Schroth Diet *which should only be carried out under the expert supervision of your Natural Therapist.*

Schroth diet

This diet is effective because it temporarily deprives the body of water, its most important constituent. The treatment is planned as follows:

First day: small quantities of liquid
1 Morning: Bowel evacuation with saline purge or enema
2 Until mid-day: only toasted bread, but as much as you desire
3 Mid-day: 250–500 grammes of cooked oatmeal or rice with prunes
4 4 p.m. until supper: 100–125 cc of warm wine or fruit juice, or alternatively
5 7 p.m.: gruel made from rice, semolina or barley
6 Bedtime: cold body pack

Second day: *large quantities of liquid*
1 Until mid-day: you may eat only toasted bread or dry biscuits
2 Mid-day: 250–350 grammes of cooked oats with apple sauce
3 4 p.m. until bedtime: you may drink 500 cc of tea, fruit juice or wine
4 During the evening: application of a cold body pack

Third day: *dry diet*
1 No liquids are permitted during this stage of the diet. You may suck a few slices of lemon if you are very thirsty, although should you feel weak, you may drink black coffee
2 You may eat toast, dried prunes; a cold pack will be applied during the course of the evening.

This regime is carried out as follows: on Mondays and Thursdays the 'first day' treatment is given, on Wednesdays and Saturday the 'second day' treatment is used, and on Tuesdays, Fridays and Sundays the 'third day' instructions are carried out. The cure lasts, on an average, for three weeks and during that time you will generally wash your mouth frequently with tepid water to bear the thirst better.

The Schroth Diet is recommended for a number of chronic conditions, e.g. diseases of the joints, the skin and the liver, and for chronic catarrh. The Schroth cure may be particularly suitable for people who tend to retain fluid in their tissues. The treatment can be varied and can be made less drastic; for instance, the enema and the purging can be omitted, and the body pack can also be left off.

Milk diet
While the Schroth diet eliminates fluid from the body through purging, and through encouraging perspiration by the application of body packs, and at the same time reduces the intake of fluids, the Milk Diet achieves elimination of fluids by stimulating the kidneys. Each day in the course of this regime you drink four glasses of milk, to which one litre of Vichy water or distilled water may be added. On this form of diet, you lose sodium chloride (common salt) through your kidneys.

The Milk Diet can be continued for four days. It has been found beneficial in cases of heart failure with retention of fluid (oedema), but it is also suitable for inflammation of the skin (dermatitis) which is associated with 'weeping', that is, the oozing of fluid.

Milk is useful not only to stimulate kidney activity, but also to inhibit bowel action and therefore is used with great benefit in cases of diarrhoea (unless the patient is unable to digest milk). Milk can be made more digestible by adding to it a culture of the lactic acid bacillus, and then incubating it at 55°F (13°C) for six to twelve hours. The same result can be achieved by adding lactic acid, drop by drop, to boiled skimmed milk (up to 45 drops to a pint). Buttermilk, the fluid left over after the milk fat has been removed, also helps cases of diarrhoea and, like milk, is a stimulus to the kidneys.

Grape diet

Whereas milk contains protein, carbohydrates, fats and mineral salts, grapes are rich only in sugar. They also contain certain acids and traces of mineral salts. Eating about four pounds of grapes per day (including the skins, after they have been thoroughly washed to remove the effects of spraying, and also eating some of the pips) for several weeks has been of remarkable benefit. People who had been suffering from a variety of complaints, including those of the liver and joints, have reported great improvement and generally feel that their bodies have been cleansed. Their kidneys and bowels are stimulated to eliminate waste and toxins. The Grape Cure is one of the dietetic treatments which help the whole body and which tend to restore your health.

Fasting on water and fruit juices

In Natural Therapy, the fast is the most dramatic way of making a change in dietetic habits. Apart from the emotional response, the physical effects vary from person to person. The results of fasting have been measured from time to time, and one such study, carried out by two medical scientists, examined the weight losses and changes in the various constituents of the body.[23] The subjects were 58 female and 18 male patients and the duration of the fast extended over more than 14 days. There was a rapid loss of weight in the first two weeks. Amongst the women, the highest figure was that of a woman of 51 who reduced her original weight of 117·4 kg by 11 kg (1 st 10 lb). The lowest figure was shown in the case of a woman of 34 whose weight went down from 122·1 kg by only 1·34 kg (3 lb). On average, men lost more weight than women during the first two weeks; after that, the mean losses for the two sexes were similar. The differences were attributed to different amounts of water excretion by the kidneys, but were also explained on the basis of different losses of physical activity. Patients showed different losses of the mineral potassium. This should be supplied during a fast. It can be given in fruit juices or as potassium salt.

Another scientific study, carried out on very fat people, found that no harmful effects were noted during the phase of initial rapid weight loss, and that there was prompt improvement in people who had serious respiratory or cardiac conditions. Common early side-effects were mild headache, occasional nausea and some nervous tension. People became less fit physically, but young ones maintained their vigour better than older patients. Sleep patterns were not affected, but sensitivity to cold was increased. The blood pressure dropped after the third and fourth week, and with this drop came a rise in pulse rate and a feeling of weakness leading to a sensation of faintness in some patients. The level of uric acid rose, causing attacks of gout in two patients.

Starvation was considered to be a strain on the heart, and a drop in blood pressure was thought to be dangerous to people who have recently suffered from a heart attack (myocardial infarction). Other people who were not thought suitable for fasting included those with a history of anaemia, liver disease, or inadequate circulation of the heart (coronary insufficiency manifest in attacks of angina pectoris). The sufferers from gout required the addition of protein.

When blood pressure dropped, patients were given food. Vitamins were required throughout. Three men developed anaemia in the second month (the experiment lasted sixty days).[24]

These experiments not only provide a Natural Therapist with some valuable information, but also highlight the difference between Natural Therapy and the conventional medical approach. The Natural Therapist distinguishes between fasting and starvation. There is no therapeutic *starvation*, according to Natural Therapy; there is only therapeutic *fasting*. This difference has been explained in the following terms: 'To *fast* is to abstain from food while one possesses adequate reserves to nourish vital tissues; to *starve* is to abstain from food after reserves have been exhausted so that vital tissues are sacrificed'.[25]

While the conventional physician sees a reason for withholding food only in cases of obesity, the Natural Therapist sees, in fasting, a most potent way of giving the body a chance of recovering from the disequilibrium which disease in general represents. The loss of weight is only incidental, although it figures prominently in cases of overweight. To the Natural Therapist, fasting means giving the organism a rest so that repair work can be carried out. Digestion puts a strain on the stomach and the intestines, on the liver, the pancreas and on all the glands which deal with the assimilation of food. The work load is slowed down during abstinence from food, which means a rest also for other functions of the body, such as respiration and nervous activity. At the same time, the mind is at rest – provided the surroundings are peaceful.

The experience of a fast can be of vital importance in your life. It can be a turning point in your attitude towards values; you can recognize and correct your tendency to over-eat, to rely on alcohol, smoking, tea and coffee. This can be the time when you come to accept responsibility for your health. Fasting is a time for stocktaking.

A patient who is frightened of the effects of fasting, or who is surrounded by well-meaning people who warn him against abstinence from food, saying that it will be dangerous to his health, cannot benefit from a fast. Therefore, fasts are often taken in a home where other patients are having the same experience, and where the staff are experienced in handling the treatment.

Under the guidance of an experienced Natural Therapist, you should feel safe and assured that the fast will be correctly terminated.

The fast is a cleansing process which may be experienced in the following way: your therapist interprets the bad breath and the coated tongue which are always present at the beginning of the fast as evidence of toxic eliminations. You are not hungry after the first two days; but you may feel sick and may actually vomit or have diarrhoea – further efforts on the part of your body to get rid of unwanted matter. You may complain of a headache – a manifestation of your toxic condition.

Gradually your appetite returns, the tongue clears and your breath becomes sweet: then the fast can be broken. During the fast, you should be allowed to rest as much as you desire. You should be comfortably warm; lukewarm sponges of your body and mild sun baths are helpful.

In an article on regeneration during a fast and while taking juices, Dr E. Heun has summarized the results of many investigations. He holds that destruction of unhealthy tissue through fasting must precede the building-up of sound cells through the taking of whole-food. Heun has classified the various tissues with regard to their capacity to regenerate: the cells of the blood and lymph, the bone marrow and lymphatic organs re-form quickly, so does the liver cell and those cells which line the inner organs, as well as the elements which form the skin. Muscle and nerve cells show much less capacity for regrowth; the cells in the brain do not grow again after they have been destroyed. During a fast, shrinking occurs in the above order of regeneration, leaving the most valuable tissues intact. Substances which are released during the death of cells stimulate the growth of new cells. This constructive process is initiated during a fast, leading to rejuvenation of the whole organism, but with advancing age, the power of regeneration diminishes.

Heun has traced the changes of the cells in the blood through the various stages and has followed their defensive actions against the toxins in the body throughout the fast. He attributes to the lymph a scavenging role. The skin looks younger after the fast, as its circulation has improved. The inner linings of the body take part in the cleansing process which is visible on the tongue, but is also evident in the intestinal and urinary tracts from the appearance of mucous secretions found in the stools and in the urine. There is regeneration of the thyroid gland, the ovaries and the testes, as well as in other parts of the body which are concerned with regulation of vital processes. At the end of his article, Heun discusses 'psychocatharsis', a spiritual regeneration, a 'digestion' of pent-up emotional waste.[26]

Fasting is beneficial in acute and in chronic disease. Any acute condition – a cold, an attack of bronchitis, of tonsilitis, any of the children's diseases such as measles – is best treated by a fast; that is, by giving only water or fruit juice to the patient. In this way the body recovers without having to cope with the toxic side-effects of such drugs as aspirin, or having to waste energy on the digestion of food. In fact, the natural instinct, when acutely ill, is to abstain from food. A sick animal does not eat when ill. In cases of chronic disease the Natural Therapist has to assess the patient's ability to respond bodily and mentally to fasting.

Many sufferers from such chronic diseases as rheumatoid arthritis, bronchial asthma and inflammation of the kidneys, benefit from a well-conducted fast. Patients who are unsuitable, from whom no response can be expected, are the very young, the very old and those who suffer from some debilitating disease such as cancer, or a chronic disease of the nervous system. In cases of gastric and duodenal ulcer, fasting may precipitate a haemorrhage and is therefore too dangerous.

The fast is broken by introducing the next grade of the natural dietetic stimulus: the raw fruit and raw vegetable regime.

Raw fruit and vegetable diet
After a fast, a diet consisting of raw fruits and raw vegetables is the next step in the stimulation of the body by dietetic means. Raw fruit and vegetables contain enzymes (elements which bring about necessary chemical changes in the body) which are destroyed by cooking and processing. As Shears has pointed out: 'In order to help furnish the body with the elements which it needs,

they must necessarily be obtained in organic life-containing form as in raw vegetables and in particular in the form of fresh vegetables and fruit juices.'[27]

Fresh fruit and vegetables also contain, in concentrated form, vitamins needed by the body. These are related to one another; therefore the taking of single vitamins can easily upset the balance. Fresh fruits and raw vegetables are alkaline-producing foods, since they form alkaline residues (ashes) and, as such, they counter the acid-forming foods such as meat, eggs, fish, cheese and game. Sugar and flour are also acid-forming. These acid-forming substances are taken to excess by many people, and the raw fruit and vegetable diet acts as an antidote. Natural Therapists believe that, in order to keep well, we need a surplus of alkaline-producing foods and that people who follow a conventional diet suffer from an upset of their acid/alkaline balance.

A raw fruit and raw vegetable diet may consist of the following items: for breakfast, muesli (oats soaked overnight, mixed with a grated apple and a little lemon juice and nut cream); for lunch and for supper, raw vegetables, nuts, olive oil. Dried or fresh fruits are added to the salads.

The patients of conventional physicians are only rarely given the benefit of this type of diet, as medical training does not provide the student with the necessary conception of a sick body responding favourably to the stimulus of a raw fruit and raw vegetable diet. To the ordinary doctor, the overriding dietetic concern is the calorific need, and the supply of the various elements (protein, carbohydrates, fats, vitamins and mineral salts) in sufficient quantities.

Dr D. C. Hare of the Royal Free Hospital in London took an exceptional step in 1936 by feeding patients suffering from osteoarthritis, acute rheumatoid arthritis, chronic rheumatoid arthritis, and 'muscular rheumatism', on one pint of milk, raw fruit, raw vegetables and Bircher–Benner Muesli made with 90 gm (3 oz) of cream. There was a remarkable improvement, a relief of pain and, in eight out of twelve patients, the joints became less stiff and less swollen. Alas, after only two weeks Dr Hare added eggs, cheese and meat.[28]. Later, the trial was repeated by Drs Hare and

Pillman-Williams on six patients suffering from rheumatoid
arthritis; five of them benefited although the sixth disappeared.[29]

Unlike a physician such as Dr Hare, a Natural Therapist, when
applying the dietetic stimulus, is not guided by a diagnosis or by
the concern to meet a patient's calorific or nutritional needs. He
observes the response and, in many cases, keeps the patient on a
reduced diet for weeks and months, with excellent results. He is
encouraged by the reports published in scientific medical
literature which confirm the fallacy of considering the human
person in terms of a combustion engine.

A striking example has been given in Sweden. Twelve men,
aged 20 to 50, walked 50 km (about 31 miles) per day for ten days
while their diet was restricted to mineral water, apple juice, orange
and grape juice, and freshly prepared carrot and red beet juice.
They also took vitamin and mineral tablets. Each man's total
daily calorific intake was 340, whereas his calculated needs would
have been well over 3,000. In spite of this 'deficiency', they
remained perfectly well.[30]. During a longer period, extending
over several months, a Japanese doctor proved that he and his
wife could maintain excellent health on raw whole rice, raw
vegetables and a little fruit.[31]

Full diet
(a) *Essential components* After you have been living on a
restricted diet and have eliminated toxins, the Natural Therapist
will proceed to build up a diet to satisfy your body's permanent
needs. Depending on your case, the full diet may be prescribed
sooner or later in the treatment. Many people who are not fit for
a strict diet because they are too old or too young, or those who
are not suffering from a serious condition which would justify
a drastic change, start with a full diet. But what is a full diet to
one person, who maintains his weight on it, is an eliminative diet
to another. The result depends on whether the digestive organs
are able to extract the necessary nourishment from the food. It is
common experience in Natural Therapy that the same amount
and combination of ingredients can lead to an initial loss of
weight in a person who, later on, maintains his weight or even

increases it. In the course of time his organs have acquired the ability to assimilate the food.

The Natural Therapist must consider an individual's likes and dislikes. To force down food which does not appeal is useless; it will not be digested properly, as the digestive juices only flow when food is wanted.

A balance of ingredients is vital. This balance is best safe-guarded by eating food grown in healthy soil and eaten whole and fresh whenever possible. We shall now briefly discuss the items which make up a full diet.

Protein. The protein should be derived from wholegrain cereals, pulses and dairy produce. Meat and fish are for those who cannot accept a lacto-vegetarian diet, even though it supplies all the necessary protein. The soya bean is a very good source of protein, as are nuts, seeds, avocadoes, almonds and yeast. People engaged in strenuous exercise require extra protein. The minimum need has been estimated to be 0·5 gm protein per kilo bodyweight.

Carbohydrate. Wholegrain, compost-grown bread, cereals such as wheat, oats, barley, rice and maize; potatoes; honey and sweet fruits such as dates, figs and grapes: these are the main sources of carbohydrate. Beetroot and root vegetables, for instance, turnips and carrots, yield further supplies and so does milk, which con-tains milk sugar. Pulses (peas, beans and so on) provide starches as well as proteins.

Fat. Cream and butter, margarine (which may be made from animal or vegetable fat), olive oil, almond oil and nuts, are the main sources of fat.

The Royal College of Physicians and the British Cardiac Society have recently warned against the customary fat con-sumption which amounts to forty-two per cent of all calories. The report insists that this high figure is an important factor in the incidence of heart disease which is particularly prevalent in Britain. The proportion of fat should be reduced to at least thirty five per cent and 'polyunsaturated' fats, such as corn and sun-flower seed oil or safflower oil should replace as far as possible the fat which is obtained from meat, butter, cream, milk and fatty cheeses. Olive oil is also preferable to cream, it can be diluted with polyunsaturated oil as a salad dressing. The Natural Therapist accepts these recommendations.

Vitamins. The following tables summarize the role played by vitamins in the body and indicates the sources of supply:

Vitamin	Sources of supply
A: Deficiency leads to diseases of the eye, the skin and the linings of internal organs. The vitamin is stored in the liver and feverish diseases can depress the store. Nitrate, used as a preservative for sausages, salami and other foods such as frankfurters, hamburgers and canned meat, also depress the vitamin A stores in the liver.	Milk, butter, eggs, liver, fish and fish oils. In a preliminary state it occurs in carrots, turnip tops, spinach, parsley, watercress, cabbage and lettuce.
B1: A deficiency of this vitamin is known to cause a great many symptoms such as fatigue, depression, dizziness, sore muscles, palpitation, chest pain, sleeplessness, loss of appetite and weight, vomiting, weakness of muscles, irregular heartbeats and low blood pressure. The body's vitamin B1 requirements are raised by the ingestion of excessive amounts of sugar. The refining of flour destroys a large percentage of this vitamin which is essential for growth and for the proper functioning of the heart, nerves and muscles.	Wholemeal bread, unpolished rice, oatmeal, milk, yeast, butter beans, haricot beans, peas, lentils, meat and eggs.
B2: This vitamin is needed to promote healthy conditions of skin, mouth and hair and is essential for the functioning of the	Meat, fish, green vegetables, potatoes, wholegrain products and brewers' yeast.

Vitamin	Sources of supply
eyes. Without this vitamin, important biochemical transformations in the body cannot take place.	
B3 (Niacin): Essential for the processes which take place in the intestinal tract, in the skin and the nervous system. Vitamin B3 is not present in white flour or in polished rice.	Wholegrain flour, unpolished rice, meat and yeast. To a lesser degree it is also present in fruit, vegetables, milk and other dairy products.
B6 (Pyridoxine): This vitamin is concerned in many processes connected with the building of body tissues. Its absence leads to such serious consequences as anaemia and neuritis. Individuals vary in their requirement of it.	Widely distributed in food.
B12 (Cyanocobalamin): A deficiency of this vitamin leads to a form of anaemia (pernicious anaemia) which is characterized by complications in the nervous system and by abnormal mental functioning. Vegans, who, as a matter of principle, abstain from all dairy produce (as well as meat and fish), are liable to suffer from vitamin B12 deficiency and have to consider taking this vitamin as a drug.	Foods of animal origin.
Folic Acid: A deficiency is responsible for anaemia.	Green vegetables, liver, meat and fish.
C: Essential for cell activity. Deficiency of this vitamin leads to scurvy, characterized by haemorrhages into the skin and internal organs. Bleeding gums are also a sign of this condition.	Fruit and vegetables, especially oranges and other citrus fruits. Also in the green leaves of vegetables and in *unheated* milk.

Vitamin

Sources of supply

Deficiency results largely from the degradation of food, and it has been estimated that there is a deficient intake of vitamin C in 54 per cent of British households during the winter months and in 25 per cent of British households over the whole year.[32]

D: This vitamin is formed in the skin by the action of sunlight, which confirms the value of sun-bathing. Vitamin D is essential for the formation of a healthy bone structure in children and for maintaining it in adults. The lack of it appears in the bent bones of the rickety child and of the adult who suffers from osteomalacia or bone softening. Extra Vitamin D is required in diseases of the gut and kidneys.

Milk, liver and egg yolk.

E: A controversial vitamin, claimed by some to be important for the proper functioning of the heart and blood vessels, but others deny that it plays any useful part in the human body at all.

Sunflower seed oil, wheatgerm oil, almonds, walnuts and soya-bean oil.

K: This vitamin is made by micro-organisms in the bowel and is lacking in the body if these normal bowel bacteria are destroyed by antibiotics. This confirms the importance of healthy bowel flora for general health, and points to one of the dangers arising from antibiotics. It is essential for the clotting of blood and for the functioning of the liver.

Widely distributed in the plant kingdom. The lacto-vegetarian diet recommended by Natural Therapists supplies it in ample proportions.

Apart from gross vitamin deficiencies, causing severe symptoms, we have to consider marginal vitamin deficiencies. These may well be responsible for decreased vitality and diminished resistance to disease. There is evidence that some people lack vitamins B1, B6 and C, and that the young and the old need extra amounts of these vital substances. As has been pointed out, the full natural diet preserves vitamins by insisting that food should be raw if possible, and certainly never over-cooked.

Mineral salts. Apart from water, protein, carbohydrates, fat and vitamins, a full diet must contain correct amounts of mineral salts. These will now be discussed.

Iron. Women lose iron with menstrual bleeding and they must therefore have extra supplies. Vitamin C facilitates the absorption of iron from the gut; thus, a lack of this vitamin can cause iron deficiency. Iron is present in meat, cereals, eggs and vegetables.

Wholemeal bread is much richer in iron than white bread, and bran is a rich source. The diet recommended by the Natural Therapist supplies enough of this mineral.

Magnesium. Your body can adjust itself to a low magnesium intake by absorbing magnesium from the bowels and by restricting its excretion in the urine. Magnesium can prevent the formation of stones in the kidneys and is of importance for general health. Many people have been found to lack sufficient amounts of it. It is removed in the refining of wholegrain cereals and in cooking of vegetables. (Thus, again, the principles of Natural Therapy are vindicated.) Magnesium is found in wholegrain cereals, nuts, raw vegetables, legumes, and also in seafood and in meat.

Calcium. As with magnesium, the body can adapt itself to a low calcium intake, but there is a grave danger in a low calcium diet, for calcium is needed for the formation and maintenance of bones and for the normal excitability of tissues. In severe calcium deficiency there is twitching of muscles. Calcium is needed (with iron) for the manufacture of blood pigment. Cereals, fruit, vegetables and milk provide calcium.

Sodium. Sodium is taken in the form of sodium chloride – table salt. As sodium chloride holds water, a deficiency will lead to a reduction in the volume of body fluids, including blood. The symptoms are fainting, weakness, dizziness, mental confusion, fall in blood pressure, and muscular cramps. As sodium chloride is lost in sweat, a sufficient supply is especially necessary in hot climates and during physical exertion. The Natural Therapist provides salt for patients undergoing heat treatment which encourages profuse perspiration – but, as we shall see later, even a cold compress can lead to perspiration, and may result in a deficit of sodium chloride in the body.

There is salt in most butter and bread, in sauces, and in preserved and canned meat. People also add salt to their food in cooking and at the table, usually more than is required by their bodies. A low salt diet is valuable in several types of diseases of the kidneys, the heart, and the liver. but people generally find severe salt restriction difficult to bear. The kidneys can protect the body from loss of salt by excreting salt-free urine, and the ordinary evaporation of water from the skin does not contain salt either. Too much salt can be harmful. especially to babies and infants (for whom there is a danger of developing high blood pressure).

Potassium. Potassium is found in most natural whole foods, for animal and plant cells are rich in it. Fruit juices are a good source of potassium. Potassium deficiency arises from losses associated with vomiting and diarrhoea. In some kidney diseases, and in wasting diseases where cells break down, potassium losses occur. The symptoms are muscle weakness, dizziness, thirst, mental confusion, and interference with the normal excitability of tissues.

Interference with mineral metabolism. The industrial development of our times has introduced harmful elements such as lead, tin, cadmium, fluoride, mercury and arsenic into the human body. These can interfere with the normal mineral metabolism, and may cause disease and deficiencies. Modern agricultural practices have led to the use of mineral fertilizers, such as lime. This may further upset the natural balance, especially of the trace elements, which play an important part in the body.

Trace elements

Iodine. Iodine is an essential component of the body, and is found in the thyroid gland. Its absence in food leads to the formation of goitre. Iodine is present in seafoods, including fish. People vary in their need for iodine. To give an excess is dangerous for people who suffer from an over-activity of the thyroid gland. Iodine and other substances are found in kelp which is made from seaweed.

Copper. Copper is present in most foods, and high intakes are absorbed from seafood, meat, eggs, nuts, fruit and cereals. Copper facilitates vital processes. On the whole, deficiency is not likely.

Molybdenum. Molybdenum is another essential trace element. It helps to prevent dental caries, and deficiency of this element in the soil makes plants susceptible to fungus infections. There seems to be a danger that the breakdown products from such plant disease can cause cancer in people who eat the diseased plants.[33]

Zinc. Zinc occurs in seafoods, meat, wholegrain products, dairy produce, nuts and legumes but not much in other vegetables. Zinc deficiency has been diagnosed in the Middle East, but not in the West. (As the result of zinc deficiency, children in Iran have failed to mature normally.) This metal is important for the production of sperm, for the growth of bones, and for certain biochemical processes. Zinc aids the healing of wounds. It is related to copper and calcium. Often, as a result of mechanization and the neglect of organic manuring, the soil has become deficient in zinc in many countries, and this fact may have a harmful effect upon human health.

In general, trace elements are refined out of cereals and, as already indicated, agricultural methods can deprive the soil of these important and not fully investigated substances.

(b) *A simple balanced diet* After having defined and evaluated the components which are necessary for a balanced natural diet, we have now to indicate how meals should be planned. Of course, people are expected to choose foods they like, and leave out foods they dislike.

When planning daily menus, note that raw fruit and vegetables (discussed in an earlier section) play a very important part in a full and regular diet. At least 50 per cent of food should consist of raw salads and raw ripe fruit.

Breakfast. Breakfast should be light since, early in the day, your stomach is not ready for much food. The food consumed on the previous day provides the energy needed for the morning; a heavy breakfast only uses up energy in digestion. Breakfast may consist of ripe fruit and yoghurt, or the muesli mixture recommended as part of the raw vegetable diet (page 39). The muesli can be made more nourishing by the addition of nuts, sweet almonds, honey, froment or wheat germ, and the fruit content can be varied. The protein in the mixture may be cream or milk, but yoghurt is better. Nut cream and almond cream are also suitable forms of protein and either can replace the dairy produce. Bran (coarse or All Bran) can be added if you are inclined to be constipated. Dried fruit, soaked overnight, and eaten with bran and yoghurt is another breakfast variation.

Lunch. Lunch should consist of a large salad meal in which leaves, roots and fruits are mixed. A dressing of olive oil and lemon juice is better than the conventional salad cream. Wholemeal bread, or some form of crispbread such as Ryvita, with vegetarian margarine and cheese, can be added or, in place of the crispbread, a potato baked in its skin. Nuts can be included as a further source of protein. The salad should be eaten as soon as the vegetables have been cut or grated, as the Vitamin C content is quickly lost when the finely shredded components are exposed to the air. Different types of graters can be used to vary texture and the mixture can include any fresh fruit that is in season and any vegetables, such as lettuce, watercress, celery, onions, leeks, tomatoes, endive, sea-kale, carrots, brussels sprouts, cabbage and red cabbage (both to be finely shredded), beetroot (not prepared in vinegar), radishes, spinach, cucumber, and avocado. Herbs can be added – either fresh (if available) or, dried. (When including cheese, note that cottage cheese is more easily digested than other cheeses and that salted cheeses are less advisable than unsalted ones. Strong cheeses are not as good for most people as mild ones.)

Supper (dinner). The third meal includes fresh fruit but also cooked food. Cooked vegetables should be taken. To supply protein, eggs and cheese can be added to the vegetables, or nut and soya dishes can be prepared. (For those who do not wish to be lacto-vegetarians, meat or fish is included.) Potatoes should be baked in their skins or steamed. Salt should be used sparingly. As dessert, fruit is greatly preferable to puddings.

Drinking. Liquids should not be taken with meals as they dilute the gastric juices, but they can be taken before or about two hours after eating. For reasons which have been pointed out, ordinary tea and coffee are not recommended; they should be replaced by herb teas, dandelion coffee, and fruit juices.

Additions
Here is a brief survey of some of the items that can be added to the standard diet to provide choice and variety and here are also warnings of the dangers to health from some of the foods.

Milk A milk diet was described earlier as a short-time measure to stimulate the kidneys and to inhibit over-activity of the bowel. We shall now consider habitual taking of milk from the Natural Therapist's viewpoint. Milk is an essential food for babies whose mothers cannot breastfeed. It is, however, harmful to some babies, especially to those who are allergic to it; in such cases, it can provoke eczema and must be replaced by substitutes. These are mainly derived from vegetables; for instance, preparations made from soya and nuts.

In the adult population, milk is consumed by many who seem to tolerate it well. It is a food which contains protein, sugar, carbohydrates and mineral salts, especially calcium and phosphorus. Sufferers from ulceration in the stomach and the duodenum are frequently advised by their doctors to drink large quantities of milk, and this often relieves their discomfort. Other people, not subject to any particular disease, adopt the habit of drinking several pints of milk a day.

There are serious dangers for such people. The Natural Therapist is concerned with balance, and drinking several glasses of milk upsets the dietetic equilibrium. Evidence of harm from drinking large amounts of milk comes mainly from investigation into the milk consumption of people who develop heart disease, the great modern killer. Some of the patients investigated had earlier suffered from ulcers in the stomach or the duodenum. In those who had been treated with a milk diet, it was found that the frequency of myocardial infarcts was double the frequency found in those who were not so treated or who had not suffered from ulcers. In a series of fourteen consecutive cases of acute myocardial infarct, nine admitted that they had been in the habit of drinking one pint of milk a day, or more.[34] A number of medical scientists investigating the blood of those who had consumed large quantities of milk found that the body had acted against milk by producing 'antibodies'. When these were present, the mortality from a myocardial infarction increased 'almost threefold'.[35] Prolonged heating of the milk (necessary in order to destroy harmful micro-organisms) seems to be an important factor in making milk harmful.[36]

Not only the heart, but also other organs can suffer from excessive milk consumption. B. Jacobson has drawn attention to the serious hazards entailed in adding daily one pint of milk to a mixed diet. This overloads the body with·calcium, phosphorus and protein. The body has to break down the protein, and this leads to the formation of oxalate, a substance which is pre-cipitated in the urine as a stone. Jacobson observed that, between 1965 and 1974, the oxalate content of stones found in men and women increased by over 50 per cent and the number of patients treated in the Leeds area in Britain increased fivefold. For this serious state of affairs, he blames the drinking of milk (shown, on average, to amount to 4·79 pints (2·7 litres) per week per person in Great Britain during 1973–4.[37]

Over-consumption of milk causes not only disturbances in the heart and in the urinary tract; the resulting imbalance leads also to disturbances in other organs. In one community which made milk almost its staple food many suffered from angina pectoris, from a tendency to congestion of the lungs, from inflammation and enlargement of the tonsils and inflammation of the middle ear. When milk was eliminated from the diet and replaced by fruits, vegetables (especially soya), nuts and seafoods, all these disturbances disappeared;[38] the fact that they were largely catarrhal supports the experience of Natural Therapists, that milk can be responsible for the formation of mucus in sensitive people.

Eggs Eggs are another good source of protein (twelve grams in a boiled or poached egg). They are also rich in vitamins. But, just like milk, eggs (in their yolk) contain a high amount of cholesterol, a substance which is involved in hardening of the arteries (atherosclerosis), and – again like milk – they endanger the heart through the formation of antibodies.[39] For these reasons, the Natural Therapist recommends only about three eggs a week. They are to be avoided by people threatened with or suffering from heart trouble and by those who are allergic to them.

Honey Honey consists of a variety of sugars, and because of its concentrated carbohydrate content should be eaten sparingly. It also contains valuable mineral salts, in which darker honey is richer than the light variety.

Soya beans Soya beans are rich in protein and fat, iron and vitamins. They should be cooked and a number of soya products are on the market. Brewers' yeast is rich in those amino-acids (the constituents of protein), which are low in the soya bean. Hence the addition of a little brewers' yeast to a soya dish makes up the deficiency.

Rice Rice is a valuable food which should be taken in the unpolished form. Nutritional losses are incurred by the conventional milling of rice, to the extent that one-third of the protein is lost by the process. By contrast, handpounding cuts out much of this loss (which, in the case of refined flour, is the loss of most of the bran).[40] As mentioned earlier, unpolished rice contains the important vitamin B1; the polished product, which has been deprived of the inner husk, is devoid of this vitamin. (Its absence in the diet leads to the disease known as beri-beri which can be cured by substituting unpolished brown rice for white polished rice.)

Sprouting grains In the process of sprouting, grains not only gain enormously in vitamin content but also supply first-class proteins. One study quotes the following impressive analysis of sprouting wheat seeds: 'Sprouting wheat seeds have been analyzed and found to contain 30 per cent more vitamin B; 200 per cent more vitamin B2; 90 per cent more niacin (vitamin B3); 30 per cent more pentothenic acid; and 100 per cent more biotin and pyridoxine (all components of the vitamin B complex) than dormant wheat seeds. During germination, vitamin C is increased by 60 per cent in cereals and germinating soya beans are so rich in vitamin C that a tablespoon of them supplies up to half an adult's daily requirements'. The same author also quotes Dr Francis Pottenger Jr, who 'found that sprouted grains and legumes provided enough first quality proteins to be classed as "complete" '.[41]

It is essential to buy seeds which have not been treated with fungicides such as mercury. The technical details of how to use wheat and rye grains (the commonest varieties) are as follows: the cleansed wheat or rye grains are used either separately or mixed in equal quantities. They are completely covered with water in a container and left overnight with a lid on. The next morning the water is poured off and the grain is left. In the evening fresh water is used to cover the grains. This procedure is continued until the sprouts are visible and have reached the length of a quarter of an inch (6 mm) (they must not be allowed to get bigger). During the process of sprouting, the grains become softer, so that they can be chewed comfortably.

The sprouting should take about three days. In the morning and evening the grains are put into a strainer and rinsed thoroughly with fresh water to remove the yeast and acidity which have developed. The sprouting grains can be eaten mixed with milk, rolled oats, and honey or sweet fruits. One to two tablespoonsful of linseed or nuts can also be added. An average daily quantity is two to ten ounces (56–280 grammes) of sprouted grains.

Seeds (unsprouted) Several edible seeds make valuable additions to the diet without having to germinate. Sesame seeds are an example. Once grown by the Romans, they are now cultivated in America, and 'the outstanding characteristic' is the high content of calcium, and of protein – 'between 19 and 28 per cent more than many meats . . . Sesame also contains an ample amount of lecithin [a fatty substance which is an essential element of the cells composing the body] . . . It is especially rich in two B vitamins . . . as well as niacin. Finally sesame is a good source of vitamin E. Sesame seeds form an alkaline rather than an acid reaction within the body.'

The seeds can be incorporated in baked foods or combined with honey, or they can be mixed into vegetable dishes. Liquified sesame seed can be made into sesame milk and can be added to many foods.

Pumpkin seeds are held by one German doctor to be a specific remedy for prostatic enlargement, which is very prevalent among men over the age of 50. This theory is confirmed by the examination of people in places (for instance Transylvania) where the seeds are eaten. These people are said to excel in virility and also to be free from prostatic troubles. An analysis of pumpkin seeds reveals a high content of phosphorus, iron, zinc, B vitamins, protein and fat (in the form of unsaturated fatty acids).[42]

Sunflower seeds are a very rich source of protein, vitamins, minerals, fats and vitamin E, and they also contain iron. They are high in fibre and thus promote the formation of bulky stools, acting against any tendency to constipation.

Avocado pears Avocado pears contain 8 per cent fat, considerable amounts of sodium, potassium, calcium and phosphorus, and some iron and copper, and they are also rich in vitamins. Not

only are they a most nourishing food, but their thick skins
protect the fruit inside from contamination by sprays.

Psychodietetics of natural therapy

The natural diet provides ample choice, which means that you
can choose your foods according to your particular taste. A
Natural Therapist must be aware of this personal factor.
Effective dietetics is incomplete if the mind is not taken into
account. Thus, psychodietetics has to be included within Natural
Therapy. 'Psychodietetics, while in itself not a science, does
provide for the interrelationship of those sciences that have to do
with psychology and nutrition. Sociology, psychology, physiology,
home economics, biochemistry, and other special fields where the
scientist is inclined to remain segregated in his research
laboratory are brought together to give practical information to
those who can utilize it.'[43]

There is a mutual relationship between the type of food which
is consumed and the mind of the consumer: a fault in nutrition
adversely affects not only the body but also the mind, and can
lead to lassitude, irritability and, in the case of severe deficiencies
of such vitamins as nicotinic acid, to insanity. On the other hand,
a faulty mental attitude, or emotional illness, can cause you to
refuse to eat wholesome food and to neglect your dietetic
requirements.

The extent to which Natural Therapy prevents or corrects
physical ailments is obviously valuable from the psychological,
as well as from the physical, point of view; for physical ill-health
causes mental suffering. If you achieve generally better health
through adopting a Natural Therapy dietetic regime, you will
feel better *as a whole person*, which means that your mental
condition has benefited from the treatment. As this form of
therapy has not been imposed upon you, you will have chosen to
change your eating habits in favour of those of Natural Therapy
and you will have the satisfaction of personal achievement if your
health improves physically and mentally. Behaving responsibly
carries its own reward.

The case for adopting the Natural Therapy regime is convinc-

ing, but people frequently resist convincing arguments and fail
to behave in a responsible way. The human mind is not only
logical and rational but also emotional and irrational. The
Natural Therapist must be aware of the emotional factors which
operate in relation to the implementation of his principles.
Psychodietetics have isolated the following factors: (1) Hunger,
(2) Appetite, (3) Habit, (4) Custom and (5) Symbolization.

1 Hunger

Hunger has been defined as a 'prime drive' in human behaviour.
In our affluent society many people hardly know the feeling of
hunger, but Natural Therapy provides them with this elemental
sensation. You feel hungry at the beginning of a fast. A
reassuring attitude on the part of the Therapist is essential to
guide you through the stage of hunger, and to prevent you from
experiencing any feelings of panic that you are suffering some
serious harm by going without food. During a low-calorie diet of
fruit and raw vegetables, with some protein such as yoghurt,
people who are used to a diet containing more calories also feel
hungry. Many of them are too fat; they must learn to bear their
hunger as the price to be paid for losing unhealthy and unsightly
fat.

Some obese people are compulsive eaters. When we first
mentioned the subject of obesity (page 24), we quoted the
definition of emotionally disturbed fat patients as people who
'have learned to turn to food whenever they become anxious or
upset'; food for them is 'the short-term panacea for all emotional
stress'.[44] A Natural Therapist can help these patients to give up
their compulsion only if he can help them to resolve the emotional
conflict which stimulates their voracious hunger, but such treatment requires skilled psychotherapy.

Paradoxically, there is a risk that the compulsive eater may
turn totally against food and become a sufferer from *anorexia
nervosa*. This is a dangerous condition, as the patients (usually
young girls who are afraid of becoming too fat) may starve
themselves to death. Unconscious guilt feelings, and the desire
for suffering or death, play a part in those whose natural hunger

is suppressed. To prescribe a fast or a strict dietetic regime for such patients would be a grave mistake, as the Therapist cannot rely on the sound instinct for life which manifests itself in normal hunger.

2 Appetite

While hunger is an elemental instinctual drive, appetite is just a tendency to eat. Earlier on, the centre in the brain which regulates a person's appetite, the 'appestat', was mentioned, and an abnormal functioning of this centre was suggested as one of the causes of obesity. Your appetite is stimulated by taste, smell and touch, as well as by the sight of food. Food must be attractive and appetizing. On no account should you feel any revulsion from it, and your individual tastes should be accepted within the framework of Natural Therapy. This means that you must be helped to replace cravings for unhealthy foods, such as sweets, and pastries made from white flour, by the enjoyment of simple, attractive natural foods, such as salads and fruits. Your appetite is further influenced by emotions; generally, you gain appetite in a relaxed and happy state and soon lose it in a state of tension, anxiety, depression or excitement. Your surroundings often determine the emotional climate, the arousal or suppression of appetite. The Therapist must be aware of these facts and try to promote favourable conditions.

3 Habit

The reform in eating that is advocated by Natural Therapy is a reform in your habits. Eating sweets, drinking tea and coffee, over-eating in general, are in many cases the result of having fallen into bad habits. Often the fault dates back to childhood. Parents indulge their children by buying them ice-creams, candy and other unwholesome treats, when they could give them sweet fruits such as dates or grapes instead. Schools feed children on white bread and puddings made from white flour. To break away from such wrongly acquired tastes is difficult if you have become dependent on them. People have to learn to discipline themselves and not to rely on unhealthy food and drinks – on endless cups of tea and coffee to stimulate their tired bodies and minds. Once the task has been grappled with, you can experience the change as something exciting. Adopting new and healthy habits is an adventure and not a punishment. It can be exhilarating. This is the attitude which your Natural Therapist will convey to you.

4 Custom

Man is not only a creature of habit, he is also a follower of customs; what other people in his society do becomes his norm. To differ from the crowd is painful because people do not like to be conspicuous.

The Natural Therapist must consider the social factor, the customs of eating. Children, in particular, suffer if they are not allowed to share in the food at school or at children's parties. Enforcement can cause considerable harm to the children's minds, and the Natural Therapist may decide to compromise rather than to insist on wholesome food. The case of the adult is easier. He can stand up to friends or relatives, and can explain the reason why customary food is refused. But here also, the strain may be considerable, and it would certainly be wrong if, as a follower of Natural Therapy, you were to cut yourself off from your social group and become isolated.

5 Symbolization

Your Natural Therapist has to be aware of the deeper emotional reasons why people cling to faulty food habits and customs. Eating is pleasurable, and many people resent the discipline of going without certain foods as a deprivation of pleasure. The Natural Therapist can point to the pleasure of eating wholesome foods, but also, as over-eating is always harmful even though pleasurable at the time, he may have to put to the patient the alternative of the pain of illness to the foregoing of culinary pleasures. People who have been deprived of love and affection, lonely people, take to eating, especially of sweet foods, as a compensation. To them, food stands for comfort, but it can also stand for status. White bread used to be a privilege of the rich, but then it became coveted by the other classes who did not want to be left behind.

Desires for, and refusals of, food can be the expression of deep psychological attitudes. Not to conform, whether to Natural Therapy or to any other school of thought, and to disregard advice, can be an act of aggression or defiance. Food is just one of the means by which it is possible to express such unconscious feelings.

Food symbolism may be spiritual. Vegetarians insist that it is morally indefensible to kill animals for food. This conviction is, however, consistenty followed only by the vegan, who refrains not only from meat and fish, but also from eggs and milk products, and thus does not promote the rearing of domestic animals for slaughter. In a vegan diet, pulses and nuts provide the bulk of the protein. Not everyone can live on this type of food.

Conclusion

Natural Therapists have to understand a person's needs for food as an expression of his body, mind and spirit. They have to be alive to the complexities of the human personality. At the beginning of this chapter, we noted the shortcomings of the conventional scientific nutritional approach, when we quoted Dr Hall's call for a new science which considers social, political, economic and ethical factors as well as the biochemical inter-actions that are set in motion by taking food into the millions of cells in the body. Recently, American scientists who are concerned with cancer have accepted some of Hall's views and have confirmed the validity of the principles of Natural Therapists in their emphasis on wholeness of food and the avoidance of any unnecessary additions. They have warned against the dangers from cancer-causing agents in the environment, and especially from the taking of cancer-producing chemicals in foods including herbicides and pesticides.[45]

Researchers have affirmed that diet deficiencies and excesses may, directly or indirectly, cause half the cancers in women and a third of those in men. High animal fat, excessive alcohol, deficiencies in vitamins A and C, food additives and man-made food contaminants are incriminated. Over- as well as under-nutrition is also blamed (confirming the view of balanced diet advocated by Natural Therapists).

Cancer of the large bowel, a common site of the disease, was singled out for study. The report said that this was possibly caused by an 'affluent' diet, 'particularly the excessive consumption of animal fats and a relatively low consumption of fibrous foods'. Meat eaters, compared with strict vegetarians, were found to suffer two to three times the risk of developing cancer in the large bowel.[46]

The health of the bowel, especially in relation to diet, will now be discussed in detail, not only with regard to cancer but to health and disease in general.

4 Health and your bowel

Food and its fibre content: the need for roughage
A diet composed largely of refined carbohydrates is deficient in roughage, normally provided by bran and fibre. It has been found that if bran is added to the diet and if plenty of vegetable fibre is ingested, some diseases which are prevalent among civilized people can be avoided or successfully treated. As a result of a high-fibre diet the stools become more bulky and the contents pass through the gut more rapidly.

The significance of roughage has been demonstrated in a number of conditions. Cancer of the large bowel, for example, is related to diet. According to recent statistics, 10,111 people died of cancer of the rectum and colon in 1970 in England and Wales, but there is a low incidence of this disease in rural African, Asian and Japanese communities, and this fact has been related to the 'bulky high-residue diet they ingest'. However, when these people adopt a Western low-residue diet, the incidence reaches that of Europeans. It is assumed that a substance which promotes the development of cancer has less time to act on the lining of the bowel in the case of fast transit, encouraged by roughage, than when constipation is present.[1]

Apart from cancer of the large bowel, lack of roughage in food plays an important part in a condition which is very common in Western people of middle or old age: diverticulitis, which is characterized by the formation of small pouches arising inside the gut. The diverticula are liable to become inflamed, which can give rise to serious complications, such as perforation which requires an urgent abdominal operation. In cases of inflammation of the diverticula, there is fever and general malaise and the patient suffers from abdominal colic.

There are also interesting studies which connect the fibre content of the diet with the secretion of bile and with fat metabolism. Serum cholesterol, a factor in the causation of coronary disease, is much lower in adult vegetarians (who consume more fibre than meat-eaters) than it is in non-vegetarians.[2]

The bowel flora

The bowel, especially the large bowel, harbours millions of germs which form the bacterial flora. These micro-organisms perform essential functions for the well-being of their host. Their composition varies. The coli variety is not predominant in a healthy bowel.

Diets which are rich in refined carbohydrates cause an overgrowth of the coli organisms in the bowel, which in turn predispose to infections of the gall bladder, appendix, and kidneys, conditions which were earlier listed as manifestations of the saccharine disease.[3] Meat consumption also increases coli formation.

The bowel flora contributes to the synthesis of vitamin B12 which is encouraged by a vegetarian diet. A Natural Therapist uses food to normalize the intestinal flora and yoghurt, in particular, has been found to have favourable effects. Yoghurt is made by allowing milk to ferment with a culture of certain beneficial germs (lactobacillus acidophylus, lactobacillus bulgaricus, and streptococcus thermophilus), the result being a thick acidified curd. Eating yoghurt produces a predominance of the lactobacilli in the large gut which have been shown to act against harmful micro-organisms such as agents which cause dangerous bowel infections (shigella and salmonella). Yoghurt cures diarrhoea better than certain powerful antibiotics (for example neomycin). In a Canadian hospital, yoghurt fed to infants prevented the spread of an epidemic of diarrhoea[4] and this effect was confirmed by another writer, working in Britain.[5]

Not only diarrhoea, but also constipation is helped by yoghurt, and two Americans provided proof of other benefits, derived from it. They fed yoghurt and prune whip to 194 patients suffering from constipation (their average age was seventy-one, and many were diabetics). This treatment resulted not only in an improvement in their bowel action, but the yoghurt, working on the intestinal flora and, indirectly, on the whole body, cleared up skin trouble (seborrhoeic dermatitis), healed chronic diabetic ulcers, and generally improved the old people's morale.[6] Studies on animals have shown that, by producing a healthy bowel flora, it is possible to prevent the spread of toxins from the bowel into the body.

Attacks of diarrhoea and disease of the liver have been relieved by giving the *Lactobacillus acidophylus*, a constituent of yoghurt, as were attacks of migrane in eight out of ten patients by such a regime.[7] Thus, the importance of the concept of the whole man is vindicated by studies which demonstrate the significance of a healthy condition of the gut for the rest of the body.

Natural elimination
Moving the bowels is an important function. It has been shown that regular evacuation can be achieved through promoting healthy bowel flora and through a rich fibre content in food. Lack of physical exercise is another factor causing constipation, and a further cause of this common complaint is found in ignoring nature's call; as a result, people become unaware of the fullness of the rectum. This fault often dates back to childhood, when a boy or girl was not trained to visit the toilet before going to school. When the child experienced the urge during lessons, he or she was often too shy to ask to be excused. In such cases, a Natural Therapist has to re-educate the patient to become aware of the fullness of the rectum and the following yoga exercises against constipation will help.[8]

Exercise 1: (*Ghenanda Sambita II, 15, 24; III, 21, 82*)
The patient sits with his knees straight. He bends forward and touches his toes with his finger tips, at the same time opening the anus (as if having a motion); on leaning back he contracts the anus. This exercise should be carried out every day for fifteen to twenty minutes, with intervals.

Exercise 2: (*Ghenanda Sambita II, 14, 22, 24*)
The patient squats in a bath which is partly filled with water; his
knees should not touch the floor of the bath and his heels should
be pressed against the buttocks. The patient separate the buttocks
by pressing his heels apart, and thus opens the anus, at the same
time breathing out as deeply as possible. This causes negative
pressure on the rectum, and a small quantity of water enters. He
then closes the anus. He repeats the exercise a few times, thus
giving himself an enema and the bowel is then emptied.

Both these exercises, especially the second one, have to be
practised for some time before patients can carry them out well.

Laxatives should be avoided whenever possible, as they tend
to lead to more constipation after the stimulation has worn off.
Liquid paraffin should not be taken, as it absorbs fat soluble
vitamins, thus depriving the body of them. Also, some of the
paraffin gets absorbed and collects in the lymph nodes within the
abdomen where it can give rise to swellings. 'Isogel' and
'Normacol' are harmless; they induce soft, bulky stools, and the
beneficial effect of bran on stool evacuation has been
emphasized already.

If the patient's bowels do not move spontaneously, and if
neither harmless medicinal aids nor special exercises overcome
constipation, Natural Therapists may resort to the use of
suppositories, enemas or colonic irrigation. However, suppositories and enemas should not be given over prolonged periods
as they tend to abolish the natural reflex which is nature's call to
empty the bowel.

A glycerine suppository or the more drastic 'dulcolax'
suppository stimulates the bowel and clears the rectum. An
enema can be administered either with a Higginson's syringe or
preferably with a gravity douche. The enema consists of lukewarm
water or normal saline (1 tablespoon of common salt to one pint
of warm water) or of an affusion of herbs such as camomile or a
soapy solution. Enemas bring about defecation by distending the
bowel, but, as with suppositories, people become dependent on
them.

A colonic irrigation reaches sections of the lower bowel which are beyond the reach of enemas and suppositories, but the main purpose of irrigation is not just the removal of faeces but the washing out of the bowel. This lavage can improve the tonicity of the bowel wall and thus help to overcome constipation, as the bowel musculature gets stronger. Since Natural Therapists consider the elimination of toxins to be an important part of their treatment, enemas and colonic irrigations are often combined with the use of eliminative diets, particularly in conjunction with fasts, but the subject is controversial.

One Natural Therapist considers that any measures which force elimination via the bowels (and also via the skin and the kidneys) during a fast are harmful. Instead, he relies entirely on the inherent healing power within the body which, he claims, causes the bowel to empty itself.[9] Other Natural Therapists insist that enemas and irrigations form an essential part of the eliminative treatment. High enemas and colonic irrigations are also employed to relieve the spasm in the urinary canal when it is blocked by a stone, and thus facilitates natural passage of the stone. Further benefits from irrigations are claimed in inflammatory conditions of the gall bladder and of the female internal genital organs. In cases of diverticulitis, the contents of the pouches are washed out and the bowel is cleared and encouraged to contract better. The mechanical effects of the large amounts of warm water can also have a beneficial result on the bowel flora. Colonic irrigations must not be used, however, if the anal sphincter is weak, if the patient suffers from painful piles or an anal fissure or a fistula (an abnormal opening of the rectum into the skin), from any other painful anal lesion, from an infection of the lower bowel, or from a growth in the bowel.

The functioning of the bowel is intimately connected with the mind. The Natural Therapist has to be aware of this relationship and has to realize that constipation and diarrhoea may be the result of emotional disturbances, and that enemas, suppositories and irrigations may have harmful psychological consequences. While elimination is obviously important for general health, bowel-consciousness should be avoided and the idea which was prevalent in a previous generation that harm is to be expected if evacuation does not occur completely regularly (an idea which led to the abuse of laxatives) must be resisted.

Physiological and psychological factors play a part in all the organs with which the Natural Therapist is concerned. We shall now discuss the lungs, which stand for the very breath of life.

5 The breath of life

A brief survey of the role which the lungs play within the organism makes us realize their importance for our general health. These vital organs provide the body with oxygen; they eliminate the waste product, carbon dioxide, allowing both these gases to pass through their fine pores. They act as a filter, removing many harmful substances from the blood, and they store, transform and change vital chemical elements which are present in the body.

Air pollution and your lungs

In many people, the delicate structure of these organs suffers severe damage, as is evident from the following authoritative statement: 'Chronic respiratory disease characterized by productive cough and obstruction to bronchial air flow presents important social, economic and medical problems. Death rates and epidemiological studies have established it as a major cause of ill-health and death in the middle-aged and elderly, especially in this country'.[1]

An important factor in the causation of this illness is *air pollution*. A recent report on the situation in the USA reveals 'some shocking figures. . . . For it has been discovered that nearly half the non-smokers in the country have more carbon dioxide in their blood than American Federal Standards deem safe'. With regard to the poisonous gas, carbon monoxide (CO), results were obtained from the analysis of blood taken both from non-smokers and from smokers. When interpreting these findings, the fact has to be borne in mind that people develop a certain tolerance to carbon monoxide, but that in non-smokers this tolerance is lower than it is in smokers (smokers can tolerate two to four times as much CO as non-smokers). 'Under the Clean Air Act Quality Standards air is regarded unsafe if the CO in a non-smoker's blood reaches 1·5 per cent saturation after eight hours' exposure.' The research carried out at the Medical College in Wisconsin revealed that in 45 per cent of tested non-smokers this figure was exceeded. With regard to the smokers, some of their blood was 'so saturated with CO that they should not donate their blood to heart patients'. Because of CO air pollution, some big airports, such as New York's JFK, are not safe for long waiting periods for travellers with advanced heart and lung diseases. Even slightly elevated levels of CO 'can pose a big danger to infants, the elderly, or people with heart or blood vessel diseases'. Car fumes figure decisively, making Los Angeles even less safe than the larger cities of New York and Washington. However, in all three cities, 'three-quarters of the non-smokers had unsafe concentrations in the blood'. Even rural areas were far from unaffected; the inhabitants of villages in 'unspoiled' New Hampshire and Vermont showed 'surprisingly high CO levels'. The report lists the following factors as contributing to CO pollution: smoking, geographical location, occupation, meteorological conditions, exhaust fumes. Taxi drivers were found to suffer the greatest hazards, especially those who were smokers.[2]

Another report has been published about Great Britain, and its challenging title is '*Authorities "Totally Ignorant" of Pollution Hazards*'. It quotes from speeches delivered at the opening of an anti-pollution campaign, launched by the Pollution Research Bureau in London. In this report, the following pollutants of the air are discussed:

1 Sulphur dioxide
'The air in Britain today shows an increase of one million tons of sulphur dioxide a year over the level found during the 1952 smog. All that Clean Air Act has achieved . . . is to make people build higher chimneys so that the sulphur dioxide is distributed more equitably among the whole population.' This poison is blown

across to Sweden where it contaminates lakes and waterways.
London, the report declares, has the highest levels in the whole
country, with an all-time peak in June 1970. Such levels have been
shown even in the absence of smoke to be accompanied by
increased mortality.

2 Lead

'Practically all food and water is now polluted with lead, and the
content in the air is much the same as in the diet. . . . The situation
in Britain is every bit as bad as in the US, and perhaps even
worse.' Children are particularly susceptible; 'Even mild levels
cause permanent brain damage' in children under five. Behaviour
abnormalities and aggression are mentioned as the toxic effects.
The extent of this damage to health is made clear when the report
states that 'in some areas as many as 25 per cent of children are
affected'.

An average adult may accumulate 200 mg of lead in his bones,
although 100 mg in one dose would be lethal. Lead is re-
mobilized during a feverish illness, and during cortisone treatment which is frequently carried out by the modern doctor –
often, one must assume, without this danger being considered.

The harm from lead is largely unnecessary. The Natural
Therapist protests against the gratuitous poisoning which results
from lead in petrol. This poison is inhaled from the exhaust
fumes from cars and lorries.

3 Fluorine

Fluorine 'drifts for miles, and is condensed in fog', and its ill
effects are found in both humans and in cattle in the form of
dental lesions, lameness, fractures of the bones, and respiratory
distress. The report claims that with other air pollutants, 'doctors
are simply not sufficiently aware of the problems to recognize the
symptoms when they see them'. A Natural Therapist is aware of
the fluorine danger to health in general and does not share the
narrow point of view of those who are concerned only with tooth
decay in children. He therefore agrees with the Report which
condemns water fluoridation.[3]

Breathing and rhythm

A Natural Therapist encourages all his patients to practise deep breathing of clean air – which includes breathing in well-ventilated living rooms. Breathing is influenced by physical and mental tension and relaxation, and easy breathing can be promoted by the adoption of various positions: when sitting by leaning forward with hands resting on knees: when standing by leaning forward supporting the body on a firm object such as a cupboard of a suitable height.

A correct technique is important. Two mistakes are common: people breathe in a shallow rather than a deep way and, when breathing in, they draw in the abdomen, rather than expanding it. This means that they do not ventilate the base of the lungs through proper movements of the diaphragm. Correct deep breathing is carried out through the nose with the lips closed. It starts with exhaling – emptying the lungs – achieved by breathing out while drawing in the abdomen. You can assist this process by pressing your palms against the sides of your chest and then sliding the palms down, pressing them against the abdomen. After full exhalation, you will be ready to inhale. The abdomen and then the rib cage should be slowly expanded. Your hands can encourage these movements by gently pressing against the parts which expand against slight manual resistance. After full expansion, breathe out again. The movements extend from your abdomen to your chest while you are inhaling and down from your chest to your abdomen while you are exhaling. There is a pause before the next breath is taken.

Breathing is rhythmical and must not be forced. There are individual differences in this rhythm; hence the Natural Therapist has to adjust his techniques to the particular patient's requirements, making each patient aware of the important part which breathing plays in his treatment. Breathing is practised not only in cases of chest complaints but in all cases, since the person, as a whole, benefits from deep correct breathing.

Having discussed the lungs, we shall now deal with the skin from the point of view of Natural Therapy.

6 Natural stimulation and your skin

Skin – not just a body envelope

In order to appreciate the significance of the Natural treatment of the skin, we must understand what role this organ plays in the maintenance of health. Although essential as the 'body envelope' – a guard against the outer world – the skin also has its own vital functions, which are integrated with those of the whole organism. In addition, the skin is important for mental well being. A healthy skin is beautiful and attractive, and an unhealthy skin is ugly; thus the condition of the skin can make a person self-reliant or insecure. Many people who have skin blemishes feel self-conscious, embarrassed and depressed on account of their appearance, and in such cases Natural Therapy helps to provide not only better physical health but also a desperately needed mental uplift.

The functions of the skin point to the vital role of this organ for the body as a whole. The skin protects the body against mechanical, thermal, electrical and chemical injuries. It helps in the maintenance of body temperature, stores large quantities of water and salts, resists the invasion of germs, and absorbs gases and fatty substances. The skin is richly supplied with blood vessels. The nerves in the skin provide us with information received through touch, including a whole range of experiences including voluptuous sensations, itching, burning, and various types of pain. The sebaceous glands in the skin secrete a greasy substance which keeps the skin supple, and the sweat glands are of particular importance, since toxins are eliminated in perspiration.

Surface elimination

The significance of sweating for general health has been
emphasized in a paper by Dr St John Lyburn. He maintains that
'to sweat is a function as essential for human existence as eating,
sleeping and defecation. A normal healthy adult sweats nearly a
pint a day which evaporates, leaving a layer of minute waste
products on the surface of the skin'. The total area of sweat
glands is related to the total area of skin: 'the skin is the largest
organ of the body. It covers an area between sixteen and twenty
square feet, and each of us has between four and five million
active sweat glands'. If they were put together they would 'form
an opening as large as the mouth'.

Heat treatment

To promote sweating, the Natural Therapist uses heat treatment.
Heat is applied to the whole skin or to parts of it; it may take the
form of either moist or dry heat. We shall first discuss the effects
of the whole body being exposed to moist heat, and then the
effects of total exposure to dry heat and, finally, the effects of
local heat treatments.

Moist heat applied to the whole body

A steam bath provides for maximum perspiration. The temperature can safely be raised to a high level if the head is kept cool
through a special device used by Dr St John Lyburn. During such
therapeutic sweating, the temperature of the steam is 120°F
(49°C), whereas the air that is inhaled is cooled down to 26°F
(−3°C), the head being kept in a cooled compartment to maintain the temperature within the blood vessels in the brain at a
normal level. After the patient has been in this hot atmosphere,
he continues sweating 'in humidities from 95 per cent to 63 per
cent and at temperatures of 98·4°F (36·8°C). The following
results have been claimed for this method:

1 Lowering of cholesterol: this effect is of importance to patients
who have an excess of this substance in their blood; for instance,
people who suffer from arteriosclerosis.

2 Decreases of carbon dioxide and increase of oxygen in superficial venous blood: this means that sweating aids the function of breathing and is of benefit in diseases of the heart and blood vessels.

3 Removal of toxic substances and by-products from the detoxicating organs, the liver and kidneys.

4 The blood is made more fluid, making clotting less liable to occur.

5 Sweating can remove in one hour the amount of urea 'excreted by three kidneys and of uric acid by one kidney'.

6 Reduction of blood sugar.

7 Stopping of clots inside blood vessels.

8 Removal of ammonia from the tissues.

9 Removal of bile pigments and bile salts, thus relieving jaundice.

This approach claims to relieve conditions which are treated by conventional medicine with 'drugs which inhibit cell activity' and with tranquillisers and pain killers.[1]

To encourage perspiration, Natural Therapists do not use only moist heat; they also employ dry heat.

Dry heat, applied to the whole body – the Sauna
The Sauna is a dry hot-air bath which includes jets of moist air introduced for brief periods. The exposure to heat of 100–200°F (38°–94°C) lasts for ten minutes and is followed by an exposure to cool air or to cold water for fifteen minutes, and then by a rest for a further fifteen minutes. In Finland, the country of its origin, the Sauna is a national institution. It is visited at least once a week for cleansing purposes, and after strenuous exercise it is part of training for sportsmen. The Sauna has become popular in other countries, and its effects on the body have been closely studied. The change from heat to cold has beneficial effects on the heart, as it tends to regulate blood pressure. Physical fitness is increased in a way which is not achieved by the

usual forms of physical training. Through perspiration, considerable amounts of sodium, and smaller quantities of potassium are excreted. This is important with regard to the alkali/acid balance in the body. (As sodium and potassium are factors which increase the alkali component in the blood, people who lose these substances in their sweat have to replace them by taking such alkaline foods as fruit and vegetables, including salad. The proportionate loss of potassium is smaller than that of sodium, which has therapeutic significance, as sodium – the alkaline component of common salt – is often present in excessive amounts in the body.)[2]

The above study was concerned only with changes occurring in healthy young people, and its authors did not examine any sick persons. Their results point to the importance of this form of heat for attaining and retaining fitness, but as no precautions are taken with regard to keeping the head cool, the Sauna is a drastic form of treatment for people who are not fit, although it has its uses. For instance, rheumatologists have reported beneficial effects: weekly Sauna treatments are apparently of considerable help to patients suffering from rheumatoid arthritis; they tend to prevent fresh attacks of the disease.[3]

Attention has, however, been drawn to the dangers of this form of heat application. A preliminary investigation by the US Federal Trade Commission found that the rise in body temperature, blood pressure and pulse rate in the Sauna constitute a risk to elderly people and to sufferers from diabetes, heart disease and high blood pressure. There is further danger if steam baths or sauna baths are taken within an hour after eating or while under the influence of alcohol or the following drugs: anticoagulants, antihistamines, vasoconstrictors, vasodilators, stimulants, narcotics, tranquillizers. The duration of the Sauna must be strictly limited, and care taken to make sure that people do not exceed the time allowed.[4]

Local application of heat
Apart from applying heat to the whole skin, a Natural Therapist can selectively deal with parts of the body. Hot water can be

applied as fomentations, consisting of one layer of lint wrung out in hot water, covered with oil-silk or plastic material, which is in turn covered with cotton wool. In this way heat is kept in, and the lint can be renewed every few hours. Hot fomentations are very useful in the treatment of contaminated wounds (for instance abrasions), since this method removes grit and pus, and a clean healing surface is obtained.

As another local application, steam can be directed onto inflamed parts such as the nose or the anus, for the relief of pain and, in the case of piles, for the relief of congestion.

A hot arm bath is useful in angina pectoris, which is caused by narrowing of the arteries within the heart muscle. When the arteries in the arm are relaxed, the blood supply to the heart improves through reflex action.

Dry heat and moist heat (as in hot compresses), applied to the abdomen, relieve pain arising from intestinal colic and, applied to the loins, help in cases of renal pain due, for instance, to stone formation.

Many painful conditions, especially sprains and bruises, respond to alternative applications of first hot (five minutes) and then cold (half a minute) treatments.

Cold treatment

A warm skin can be the result of an application of cold air or cold water; this type of 'hyperaemia' or increased blood supply, is due to the body responding to the stimulus of coldness by producing its own heat. The Natural Therapist can make full use of this natural response, but it is important to discover how an individual's skin will react to the cold stimulus.

In order to assess this response, a writer, working at the Spa Wörishofen in Germany, where cold water treatment is carried out extensively, classified his patients according to constitutional types. The 'athletic' person can stand only infrequent, fairly strong applications of cold; the fat, short person or 'pyknic' can tolerate cold applications (especially cold compresses) well, and quite drastic treatment can be given. The slenderly built 'asthenic' needs warmth. In this last case, only a small area of skin should be exposed to the cold and only for a short time. The bloated, 'lymphatic' type also lacks resistance to cold, although resistance can be raised by carefully graded cold applications.

Apart from this classification according to physical types, differentiation has also been made according to psychological make-up. The circulation of the neurasthenic, emotionally weak person, is easily upset by cold, and hence great care is needed. The melancholic is slow to react and in this case a strong stimulus is needed in order to achieve any result. The sanguine type, on the other hand, responds quickly and may even ask for a strong stimulus, but caution is called for here, as the patient may be rash in his judgement and may over-estimate his physical stamina. The choleric, irascible type must learn to relax and, in this case, only lukewarm water is suitable. Generally speaking, it has been found that skin which is dry and hot responds well to repeated cold sponging, whereas a moist skin gives a better response to a wet compress.

In cases of heart failure and high blood pressure, drastic cold-water treatment should be avoided but, on the other hand, such patients benefit when made to perspire, as congestion is relieved through perspiration.[5]

The texture, colour and temperature of the skin give guidance to the Natural Therapist. A very dry skin lacks sweat glands, and therefore such a patient cannot bear heat. Neither will the person who perspires heavily be a suitable subject for intensive cold water treatment, as he is frequently a neurasthenic who shows poor response. Vinzenz Priessnitz, a peasant, who was one of the pioneers of water treatment, chose the stimulus of coldness according to the patient's immediate response to cold water. Blanching pointed to a lack of response, whilst a glowing skin indicated suitability.

Apart from these general responses, cold-water applications have an effect on the following organs: when applied to the arms or the left side of the chest, they slow the heart beat but increase the output of blood from the heart. They have a soothing effect on the thyroid gland, stimulate bowel movement and deepen breathing. Cold foot-baths increase kidney activity, tend to calm the patient and thus can promote sleep; they also relieve congestion of the head by drawing blood away from it. Cold water has an effect on the nerves which supply the blood vessels, and the result is an initial rise of blood pressure which is followed by a fall, while the tone of the vessel wall can be improved by the cold stimulus. When the stimulus has been too drastic, the patient may complain of palpitation, congestion of the head, giddiness and shortness of breath.

Father Kneipp's water cure
Exercise
Father Kneipp was a pioneer of cold water treatment. His recommendations included walking barefoot in wet grass for 15 to 45 minutes a day, on wet stones for three to fifteen minutes, in recently fallen snow for three to fifteen minutes, or in cold water (which should first reach to the ankle and later to the knee) for one to six minutes. After such exercise, the patient immediately puts on dry socks and shoes. These instructions illustrate the grading of the cold-water stimulus; for in each case it must be adjusted to the person's ability to respond, and any drastic, harmful measure is avoided – a principle also valid when using the cold compress.

Compress
The cold compress consists of a piece of linen wrung out in cold water, covered by several layers of dry wool. The grading of the stimulus is achieved by varying the thickness of the moist layer, and also the area of the body in contact with the compress. Kneipp distinguished between the 'lower compress' which reaches from the armpits to the hips, and the 'upper compress' which extends from the nape of the neck to the end of the spine. In addition, he used compresses for the chest, the neck, the hands, the arms, the feet, the calves, the whole leg and the sacral region.

For a good response, the following conditions must be fulfilled: the patient must feel warm before and after the application of the compress (which is a sign that his body has responded to the water stimulus). To obtain a favourable response, the linen must envelop the particular part of the body tightly, and the woollen layers must overlap the linen. If the compress covers the chest, back or abdomen, the whole body must be kept warm by blankets, and the patient's arms must be beneath the covers. A hot bath taken before the application of a cold compress, or hot-water bottles given while the patient is in the compress, can be used to help him to get warm and he can also be given sips of hot fluids. With the feeling of warmth, perspiration sets in.

The compress is left in position until the perspiration has stopped, then the linen is removed and the patient is left in the woollen layers – for instance, wrapped in a blanket (a turkish towel can be interposed between the linen and the wool to absorb the perspiration). At this stage, many patients start to sweat again, but in a milder form. When the patient has finally ceased to perspire, the rest of the compress is removed and his whole skin is sponged with cold water, and dried. Even if there is no visible perspiration, the compress is effective and can be left on, provided the patient feels warm. Vinegar and herbs can be added to the water in which the linen is wrung out. If the patient has not reacted with a feeling of warmth within ten minutes, the compress must be removed.

The cold-water compress causes perspiration and helps to eliminate toxic substances, especially when it covers the trunk. The particular effects on individual organs, quoted from St John Lyburn's paper, give further indications for the use of the cold compress. In cases of fever, perspiration is present anyway, and the compress is easily warmed up (except when the patient complains of shivering). It assists in the elimination of toxins during a feverish illness. A combination of different compresses is frequently called for. For instance, in the case of tonsillitis, a compress around the neck can help the local inflammatory process, while a waist compress can promote elimination of toxins. A cold compress on the forehead can relieve the headache which accompanies the fever. Inflammation of veins in the leg (phlebitis) is treated with a leg compress: a thin stocking wrung out in cold water, covered by a dry thick (woollen) stocking.

Baths

Father Kneipp gave detailed prescriptions for various forms of baths. Cold foot-baths, for example, lasting one to three minutes, draw blood away from the head and chest and are recommended to relieve fatigue and sleeplessness. They can be combined with hot foot-baths to which hay flower, oat straw or malt husks may be added.

The stimulus of the cold bath can be varied according to the area of the skin immersed. The most drastic form is the full cold bath in which the patient may stay from half a minute to three minutes. Kneipp considered that this kind of bath should not be taken more often than three times a week. Partial baths, reaching to the calves, knees, thighs, or stomach are less drastic than full baths and, for inflammatory conditions especially, Kneipp advised head, eye and other localized baths.

Affusions

An affusion consists of a shower of cold water which can be applied from a watering can or a hose. The water should flow down the body, enveloping the skin and graduations are again achieved by varying the area of the body, the time of treatment and the temperature of the water.

Damp and wet sheets and dry clothes put on wet skin

In swathing, dry linen, flannel or wool is applied to different parts of the body, which have previously been sponged with cold water. The swathing is kept in position for not longer than 30 minutes and is more effective when combined with hot water. In addition, Kneipp applied wet, coarse linen sheets of various sizes directly to the skin, a more drastic treatment than the cold compress. He also advised patients to wash their bodies with cold water but not to dry the skin, as the evaporation of the water which occurs while the patient dresses in warm clothes and stays in a warm room, has an invigorating effect.[6]

Combinations in hydrotherapy

When combining cold or hot water treatments, the Natural Therapist considers the patient's constitution and the seriousness of his condition. He may, for instance, order a cold sponging of the upper part of the body on rising, followed by a rest in a warm bed for half an hour, while in the evening the patient should take a quick, cold sitz bath before retiring. Another patient with a stronger constitution may benefit from a cold, all-over sponge each morning and a full body compress each night.

Special forms of water treatment have been devised for patients suffering from arthritis and phlebitis. Here, the stimulus is directed to the arms and legs, using lukewarm or cold water for partial immersion of the limbs and also in the form of a jet of water. As a result, the circulation is improved and the patient experiences warmth, while the joints and veins benefit from the improved circulation. The whole organism gains greater resistance to infections through the training of the circulatory system. [7]

Patients suffering from high blood pressure can also be helped by hydrotherapy. Using one method, the arms, feet and lower half of the trunk are immersed in cold water for 30 minutes every day, while the temperature is raised slowly from 37°F to 42°F (3°C to 5·5°C). The patient then rests in bed for one to two hours, parts of his body having been covered with cold compresses. This regime has been combined with air baths, walking, gymnastics, breathing exercises, and other forms of physical exercise. The diet consists of wholemeal bread, milk or buttermilk, and vegetables and fruit. The blood pressure falls in a high proportion of cases. [8]

Air treatment

To the Natural Therapist, air is important not only as the source of the oxygen which we inhale, but also as a stimulus that affects the skin. Air is trapped in the clothes you wear, and so helps to conserve the temperature of your body. In addition, the Natural Therapist considers the effects which air around the body surface has on the activity of sweat glands. Clothes should be porous to allow you to perspire; cotton underwear fulfils this function better than nylon, while wool soaks up perspiration and is liable to produce excessive heat, leading to undue sweating. Such overheating of the body is followed by a chilling evaporation of the sweat and can lower the body's resistance to infection. A woollen scarf worn tightly around the neck invites such undesirable consequences.

The ground plays an important part; if, for instance, it consists of white sand, it reflects the rays of the sun and does not absorb as much warmth as dark humus ground which retains heat well. If the ground is uneven, the force of air currents is broken. Another important factor is the degree of moisture which evaporates from the ground; this, together with the air temperature, affects the functions of the skin.

The metabolism of plants is another factor; for they give out oxygen and carbon dioxide, to which are added any gaseous emanations from the soil. A further consideration is the degree of humidity. Dry, cold air is stimulating; it invigorates by increasing the metabolic rate. Whereas intense moist heat encourages perspiration, warm moist air has the opposite effect, especially if there is no wind; it interferes with perspiration and thus with the excretion of toxic substances from the skin. A sultry atmosphere tends to hinder the production of substances which make the body immune to disease. As a result, people feel lethargic and depressed and lack appetite.[9]

The Natural Therapist welcomes a change from cold to warm, and from dry to moist, as such alterations act as a stimulus which people living in even temperatures (especially if their homes are air-conditioned) tend to miss. Frequently, the recommendation is to wear fewer layers of clothing.

To sum up: the three elements, temperature, wind and moisture, with their variations, determine the effects which air has on the skin. These effects are combined in the air bath.

The air bath

People vary in their ability to stand up to cold, and the Natural Therapist must adapt air baths (like all other forms of Natural treatment) to the individual patient's capacity to respond. He must also keep in mind that the air bath not only affects the patient's skin, but also influences the lungs, since the temperature, moisture and degree of purity of the air modify the depth of breathing and the secretion from the mucus-forming glands in the bronchial tree. At the beginning patients' bodies should be only partly exposed to cool air; later the whole body should be uncovered. Air baths can be given in bed; the room may be heated, and the duration of the air bath must be adjusted to the patient's condition. Taken out-of-doors, air baths are best combined with exercises or with the playing of games.

With regard to individual diseases, there are no strict guidelines for the Natural Therapist; for, as I have shown, he is mainly concerned with the individual person's reaction to a natural stimulus. He must, however, also consider the diagnostic classification, which is fundamental in scientific medicine. Air baths with their accompanying effects on the lungs, are helpful in feverish diseases. In cases of bronchitis, the lungs benefit from an improved function of the skin, but the effect of the temperature and moisture of the air needs careful assessment. Some people's coughs get worse when they inhale cool air, others are helped. Since the skin is an excretory organ it acts in cooperation with the kidneys, and air baths are recommended in chronic nephritis. There is a further relationship between the skin and the lining of the joints; hence air baths are helpful in the various forms of arthritis. These are a few examples; the list is far from being complete. Air treatment is often combined with, and is itself an essential part of, sun treatment.

Sun treatment

When prescribing sun treatment, the Natural Therapist is guided by the intensity of the response which is to be expected. The first or mildest degree consists in a sensation of warmth which is due to an increase of blood flow. At the same time, the sebaceous and sweat glands are stimulated, but perspiration is visible only if the air is humid. Tanning occurs according to the person's ability to produce pigment. After a longer exposure the second degree of response is characterized by slight redness which is followed in the course of the next few days by tanning, and here we are dealing with a mild form of inflammation of the skin. The third degree, when the patient has been too long in the sun, consists of more intense inflammation which can go on to blister formation, accompanied by general malaise and sometimes shock and fever. A light skin is much more likely to be burnt than a dark one, and fair-skinned people are also sensitive to exposure to wind which reduces their tolerance to sunshine.[10]. Whereas an immediate adverse effect is sunburn, the prime danger of over-exposure to the sun is in the possible formation of skin cancer.

The power of the sun is greater during the morning, before it has reached its zenith and it is, of course, stronger during the summer months than during the rest of the year. When the sun is very hot, the leaves of a tree provide very good protection against an overdose, but, in any case, the head must be shaded. Reflections from the ground and from the sea intensify the effects of sun on the skin. In high altitudes the force is increased; if the ground is snow-covered, the reflection is intensified; hence exposure must be shorter. Patients can stand sun-treatment better when moving about than when resting; therefore it is a good plan to combine heliotherapy with gymnastics and games. Over-heating has to be avoided (as otherwise there is a danger of sunstroke); cold-water applications are helpful here. On the other hand, chilling is a danger when there is a cold wind, and people may have to cover parts of their bodies.

Sunlight treatment played a most important part in the years before the discovery of the antibiotic drugs which have a specific effect on tubercular infections of bones, joints, internal organs (kidneys and peritoneum, for instance), and the skin. These conditions responded dramatically to sunlight. The pioneer of this treatment was A. Rollier, working in Switzerland. Although there is no further need for his sunlight cure for 'surgical' tuberculosis, the Natural Therapist of today can draw inspiration from the changes in people's health which Rollier and his associates achieved; for patients whose bodies had become emaciated through a tubercular infection were transformed into well-nourished, strong people. The sun cured not only their tuberculosis, but brought about excellent general health.

Apart from stimulating the blood vessels and glands of the skin, the sun stimulates the underlying muscles. Other organs also benefit, partly because vasodilation in the skin leads to a reduction in congestion elsewhere. The blood supply to the organ which is affected by disease is of importance, for a highly vascular tissue (lungs, peritoneum) reacts more violently than a less vascular structure (e.g. the lining of a knee joint).[11] Rollier further stressed effects on the nervous system, effects starting from the nerve-endings in the skin and continuing by reflex action to other parts of the body, and generally stimulating the metabolism. The ultra-violet rays of the sun also have a bactericidal action; hence sunlight acts as an aseptic and antiseptic treatment for wounds.

Ultra-violet light enables the body to produce vitamin D. Research indicates that the short-wavelength (ultra-violet) radiations of the sun spectrum, not absorbed by the skin, are mostly absorbed by the blood, whereas only 20 per cent of the red and yellow rays and only one per cent of the blue and violet rays pass through the skin.[12]

Whether the sun has a direct effect on the formation of blood corpuscles or whether the effect is indirect, beneficial results in cases of anaemia are well-known. The rays of the sun also lead to absorption of fluid (exudates) in joint cavities, in the peritoneum, and in the pleural cavity. Abscesses heal, repair takes place in previously damaged structures such as joints and bones, and the patient loses his pain. Under the influence of the sun, body temperature rises and, if the treatment is too drastic, nervous excitement and sleeplessness may ensue.

Apart from these physiological effects, the sun affects the mind. People enjoy sunbathing and its bracing effect combined with cool air; under this treatment children lose their fretfulness, and both children and adults feel cheerful. Rollier maintained that sun-bathing is 'the finest stimulus'.[13]

Rollier recommended the following technique for sun baths: they are given three times a day and are graded. On the first day, only the feet are exposed, for five minutes; on the second day, the legs are in the sun for five minutes, and the feet for ten; on the third day, the thighs are included for five minutes; the legs now receive ten and the feet fifteen minutes' sunshine. As further areas are uncovered gradually, the whole body up to the neck benefits from the sun. The patient's disease, his general health, and his ability to produce pigment form the guide-lines.

Cases of pulmonary tuberculosis, of peritonitis and of heart disease must be treated with particular caution.

(When artificial sunlight with an ultra-violet mercury lamp is used, Rollier's technique can be followed, but the gradual exposure is not essential). Many patients can stand the sun on the whole body from the beginning of the treatment, provided the sun is not too hot and the head is shaded.

The treatment can be given in low altitudes, and the fact that the sky is overcast does not exclude radiation effects. However, the treatment in low altitudes has certain disadvantages; for, when there is a high degree of humidity, the heat in the summer months is more depressing than in higher regions, and seasonal variations with fewer sunny days have to be accepted. On the other hand, there is the advantage that the patient's body does not have to adapt itself to drastic changes, and this factor is particularly important in cases of diseases of the kidneys and heart and in excitable people. Psychological benefits do not depend on the altitude.[14]

Keeping in mind that debilitating diseases, especially tuber-culosis of the lungs and heart disease, are as a rule not suitable for sun treatment (as the necessary response cannot be expected), heliotherapy remains a valuable asset to the Natural Therapist. Skin conditions such as some vulgaris and psoriasis benefit from the sun, and some cases of neuritis including sciatica also react favourably. Apart from such local effects, the Natural Therapist values heliotherapy for its general tendency to invigorate.

7 Posture, exercise and relaxation

Your spine

The Natural Therapist not only instructs you about diet, about various applications to the skin, and about how to pay proper attention to breathing and the health of the bowels; he also teaches you how to use your body from a mechanical point of view. This re-education is of vital importance for the person who has 'forgotten' the correct way to stand, walk and relax. Matthias Alexander was a pioneer in this field; his pupil, Charles A. Neill, summarized his teachings in a booklet entitled *Poise and Relaxation*.[1] Neill pointed out that 'more and more people today suffer from poor posture', a factor which leads to faulty co-ordination of movement, and hence to tension. He cited a number of factors which are responsible for this state: anxiety, imitation of parents' habits, illness, and injuries. Whatever initially causes wrong posture, a habit is formed which persists, and he reminded us of some of the consequences: 'A wrong way of standing can lead to aching legs and backache, so too can bad habits in sitting, walking and lifting.' Apart from the direct effects upon our muscles, there are more remote effects on our general health, for instance, leading to faulty breathing and strain.

Good posture is fundamental and consists in the correct relationship of the vertebrae and the head. It gives us poise and is essential for physical attractiveness. The following two drawings help us to understand the mechanics, and Neill's comments provide an excellent explanation:

1 'The spine is not straight and should not be straightened. The curves of the spine are for your protection.

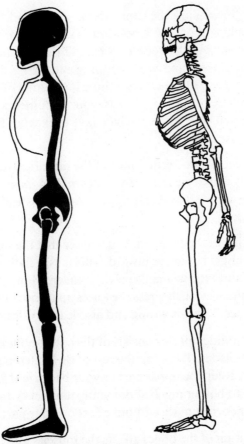

Your spine is a series of curves, all of them important and all of them affecting posture at every point in your body.

2 'The spine is the core of your body, not just something inserted at the back. Only in the upper part of the back do the bones come away from the middle line. It may help if you think of the spine as a coiled spring, which should assume its full length – neither compressed, nor stretched, but released.

3 'The chest is made of curved bones – ribs – which move on the twelve spinal bones of the upper back. An overcurved or over-straight spine will restrict your rib movements and therefore your breathing.

4 'In the lower back the bones are very large and strong, with good thick pads of gristle between as shock absorbers. Yet it is here that most 'disk' troubles occur. This is because so many people bend the spine when stooping and lifting, rather than bending the big hip and knee joints. If this area of your spine is too hollow, or curved inwards, your abdomen will protrude. If you flatten your spine you will have backache. The curve must be just right.

5 'Note the big powerful joints of the hips. Feel them on your own body. They are much lower down than most people imagine. Bend from there, also bending your knees, instead of curving your back.

6 'Looking at the skeleton, you will see that the thigh bones are not straight. They curve inward. This is especially so in a woman, since the woman's pelvis is wider. Many people, because of this, unconsciously press the knees apart because they feel knock-kneed. This is wrong and also leads to strain.

7 'The shoulder girdle consists of the collar-bones and the shoulder-blades. They join the rest of the skeleton at the top of the chest. Keep the upper part of your back right and you will not need to bother much about your shoulders – they will fall into their correct place without effort on your part.

'The position of the bones affects the muscles and ligaments attached to them. The postural muscles hold the body up against gravity.'

Neill applied knowledge of anatomical principles to teach correct standing, sitting and walking.

Standing, sitting and walking
Standing

Three pictures serve as illustrations: two faulty extremes which he termed 'too slumped' and 'too braced', and one which is 'just right'. In the slumped position, the muscles do little work and there is strain on the ligaments that hold the bones together, the curves of the spine are exaggerated, the pelvis is tilted forward,

and the abdomen is sagging. The lower part of the back is too
hollow, causing strain and fatigue.

In the second faulty position, the muscles are too contracted.
The bracing of the shoulders backwards leads to tension in the
muscles of the shoulder girdle, which results in stiffness and pain.
The pushing out of the chest prevents full rib movement and this
fault restricts breathing. The holding in of the stomach interferes
with the abdominal part of respiration. The 'tucking-in of the
tail' makes for tension in buttocks and thighs, going down to the
feet.

You are advised to check the correctness of your posture by
looking into a long mirror, or even two mirrors. In this way,
you can train yourself to adopt the right stance. The feet should
be in line, just slightly off parallel. The body's weight is spread

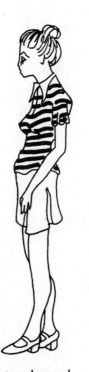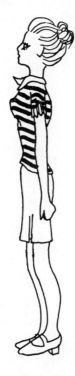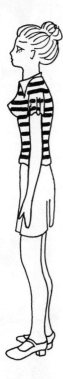

too slumped   too braced   just right

evenly over the whole surface of both feet (hence no high heels). The feet are soft and relaxed, the toes uncurled and not gripping the floor. The legs are straight, but not braced back. The whole body gently expands, the spine is straightened, the arms hang easily, the ribs move with the abdomen during rhythmical breathing. All the joints are free, and the whole body feels light. After correct posture has been mastered in the standing position, you can learn how to sit correctly.

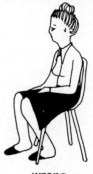 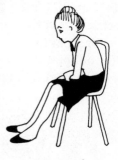 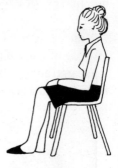

wrong   wrong again   right

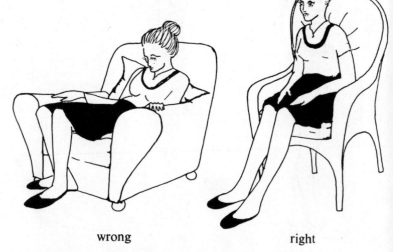

wrong   right

A firm high-backed chair is preferable.

Sitting
In sitting, as in standing, slumping must be avoided. The spine should be straight without being stretched, the shoulders should be neither braced nor drooping, making breathing effortless. The feet should be on the floor, slightly apart so that there is no tension in them or in the calves, thighs or buttocks, and the hands should rest lightly on the thighs. Illustrations of a woman sitting in a wooden chair and of another in an armchair show the faults of posture which may be encouraged by a faulty armchair; the other pictures demonstrate the correct way to sit.

Walking
The upright posture, which keeps the body in correct alignment while standing and sitting, should be maintained when walking. Neill stressed the need to balance the head. the neck muscles. and the spine, with the head held level, the eyes looking straight

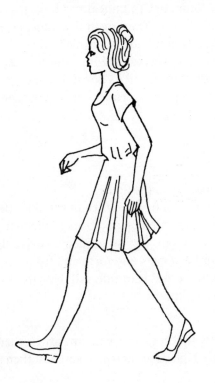

ahead, and the chin neither tucked in nor jutting out. The body
should be upright but not braced, and the pelvis should not be
too far forward, as such a tilt upsets the proper balance, causing
backache. Any swaying from side to side and bobbing up and
down should be avoided. When walking with the right posture, a
person will be aware of the free movement of hips, knees and
ankles.[2]

Apart from following Matthias Alexander's system, the
Natural Therapist encourages his patient to carry out exercises
to keep the body supple. An account of such a system now
follows:

A system of exercises

The system which has been selected aims at keeping healthy
people supple and at enabling the sick to regain mobility and
thus improve their general health. Thirteen exercises have been
compiled by Kenneth Crutchfield and form part of a wider
discussion on Natural Therapy in the home. He recommends
that the exercises should be performed slowly at first, and then
more quickly, as the person gains strength. They 'are calculated
to put the body through all its normal actions',[3] and are carried
out while standing, lying, crouching on hands and knees and,
again, while standing.

Standing

Exercise 1

Position yourself as in the figure.

(a) Rotate your head from your right shoulder down and forward
to the left shoulder, then up and back to the first position. Then
reverse the movement. Repeat sequence twelve times.

(b) Rock your head back and forth and from side to side and turn
your head fully from side to side. All these movements can be
repeated twelve times.

Exercise 2

(a) Standing with feet apart swing one arm (other arm on hip)
from shoulder high down across your chest then upwards passing

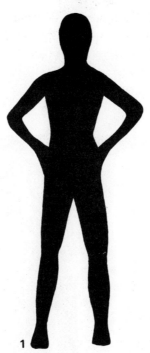

1

your face making a circle back to the original position. Repeat twelve times. Also repeat with other arm.
(b) With one arm back in line with your side (the other on your hip) swing forwards, upwards and back, making a complete circle. Repeat twelve times. Repeat with other arm.
(c) Repeat exercise with both arms together.

Exercise 3
(a) Bend your trunk from the hips (do not strain beyond your capacity), then move your trunk down to the right, across to the left and back to the original standing position repeating this six times.
(b) Then move your trunk forwards and rotate it to the right, backwards, across to the left and forward again. Reverse the direction and repeat up to twelve times. To increase the benefit of this exercise, carry out the movements with arms raised above your head.

Arm Swing

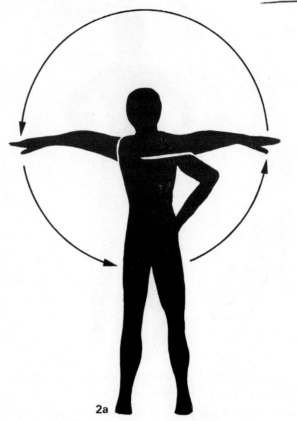

Squat

2a

Exercise 4

Start in the standing position with your hands on your hips and feet parallel but slightly apart. Then bend the knees and hips, lower your heels to the floor, extending your arms for balance, and squat with your pelvis close to your heels, the shoulders being above your knees. Repeat twelve times. To make this exercise easier, hold on to a bed-rail or to a heavy article of furniture with your hands.

Exercise 5

Stand with your right hand on a bed-rail or chair-back. Kick your left leg upwards and backwards fully with a swing making an ellipse, then sideways, forwards, sideways, back and down to the

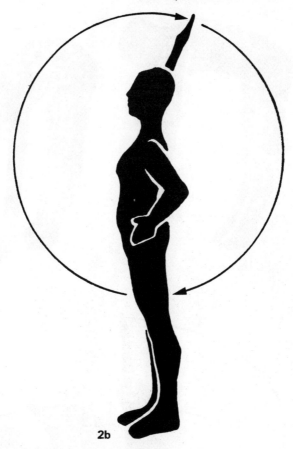

2b

starting point. Then reverse this from the back, round to the front and downwards. Repeat all movements from six to twelve times.

Exercise 6
This exercise is for the feet, and you should begin with your hands on your hips or supported for balance:
(a) Rise and fall on your toes.
(b) Rock your ankles from side to side.
(c) Stand on your heels, raising the toes.
Repeat these exercises up to twelve times or more.

As a variation of these foot exercises, place the ball of your foot

Mud Bader

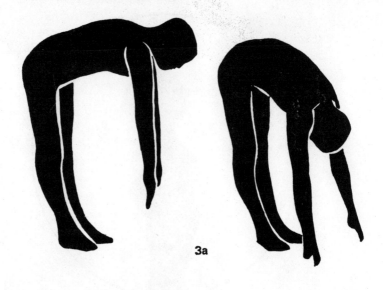

3a

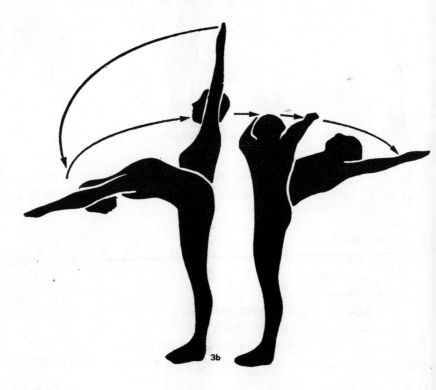

3b

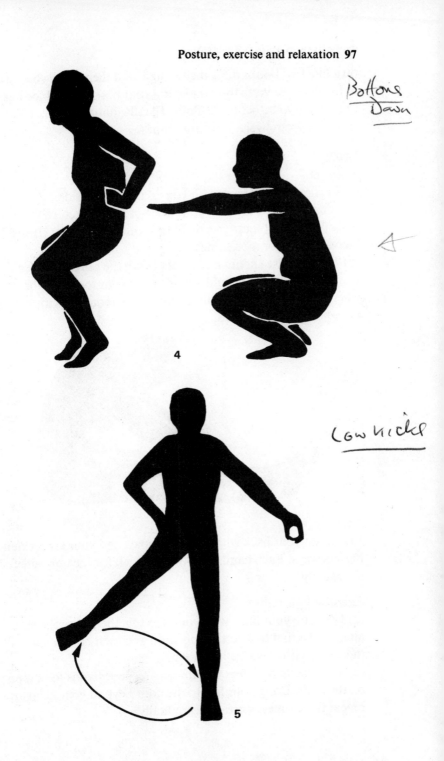

Bottoms Down

Low kicks

4

5

on a block or books three inches high, and then lower your heels to the floor. Reverse this by placing your heels on the block and then lower your toes to the floor. Finally, jump up and down on your toes from twelve to twenty times.

Lying
Exercise 7
(a) Lie flat on your back with your arms at your sides. Sit up, bending forwards towards your knees, and then return to the lying position. Repeat this three times and, as you get stronger, increase to six or more times.

(b) This exercise should be repeated with the arms extended above your head, and you should aim to reach your toes with the hands when bending forward. This modification requires extra strength and should not be forced.

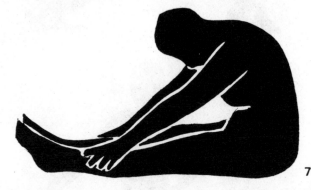

7

Exercise 8
Lie flat on your back with your legs apart and your arms extending sideways. Each hand should then reach for the opposite foot, alternately.

Exercise 9
(a) Lying on your back with your legs together, raise the legs alternately, first to a vertical position and then beyond and above the head, with knees kept straight.

(b) Then move both legs together, using your hands for support on the floor. Bring your feet to the floor beyond your head and repeat three times, increasing gradually.

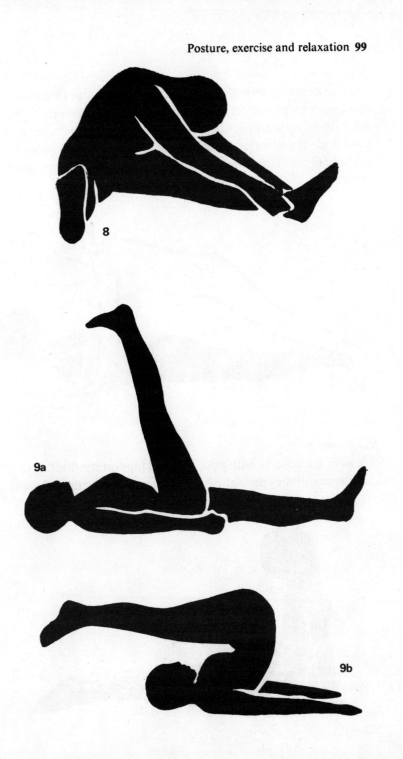

Exercise 10

Lie face downwards with your hands on the floor at shoulder
level, your trunk and legs straight and rigid, and your toes on the
floor. Press up with your arms until they are fully extended and
your body is supported on both toes and hands. Repeat this
exercise three to six times, and up to twelve times as your strength
increases.

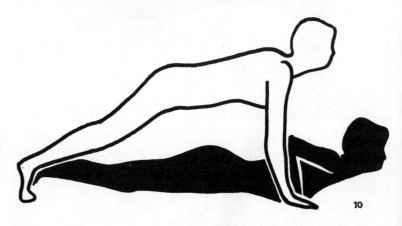

10

Exercise 11

Lie as in Exercise 10 with your legs and hips on the floor. Extend
your arms till they are straight, thus raising your trunk. Repeat
six times.

TORSO TONER

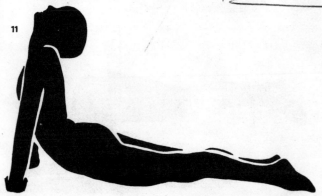

11

Nose Dive

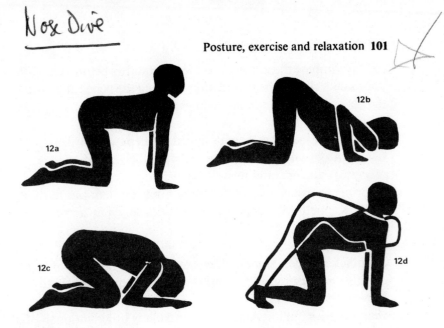

On hands and knees
Exercise 12
(a) Crouch on your hands and knees with your arms and knees perpendicular and your spine horizontal.
(b) Then bend your arms and lower your shoulders to the floor level, while keeping the hips high.
(c) Keep your shoulders low, gliding back until you are sitting on your heels. Raise your shoulders and hips once more to return to the original position (a), and repeat the exercise six to twelve times.
(d) Then recover the first position and raise and lower the lumbar spine, rocking your pelvis up and down twelve to twenty times.

Standing again
Exercise 13
(a) This exercise for pelvic rocking can be carried out either as in Exercise 12(d) or in a standing position with your feet apart and your hands on your hips as a guide to the movement. Hollow your back deeply and then straighten it, drawing the abdomen in. Then, with your legs and hands in the same position as before, and your trunk erect, rock your body from one leg to the other, repeating twelve to twenty times.

(b) To combine the above movements, stand as before, but with your knees slightly bent, and after relaxing the pelvic area, rotate the pelvis in the 'hula-hula' manner. Repeat this exercise twenty times.

The above exercises were designed to keep the body supple, but in an age when people spend most of their time sitting in offices or cars, or standing at the bench in a factory, a more vigorous approach may be required. Such a system was devised by Dr Kenneth M. Cooper and was termed by him 'aerobics'.[4]

Aerobics

Aerobics includes, among other exercises, running, swimming, cycling and jogging, and constitutes a programme to help to prevent the 'national disaster' of heart disease from which 'every year, nearly a million Americans (and many other nationals) die', and which now effects younger people and women more than it did in the past. It has been claimed that this programme lessens the chance of prematurely developing coronary heart disease or related vascular ailments and that it makes people physically and mentally alert.

The training claims to have the following effects:

'1 It strengthens the muscles of respiration and tends to reduce resistance to air flow, ultimately facilitating the rapid flow of air in and out of the lungs.

'2 It improves the strength and efficiency of the heart, enabling more blood to be pumped with each stroke. This improves the ability to more rapidly transport life-sustaining oxygen from the lungs to the heart and ultimately to all parts of the body.

'3 It tones up muscles throughout the body, thereby improving the general circulation, at times lowering blood pressure and reducing the work of the heart.

'4 It causes an increase in the total amount of blood circulating through the body and increases the number of red cells and the amount of haemoglobin, making the blood a more efficient oxygen carrier.'

Exercise charts are available for different age groups, but an initial physical examination, especially of the heart, is essential, in order to make sure that a person is fit for the training. People are urged to stay within their tolerance when exercising and to warm up at the beginning and cool down at the end. Regularity is essential in order to build up physical fitness, and Dr Cooper's book provides useful instructions regarding the distance to run, swim or cycle, or the length of time to be spent in stationary running during the sixteen weeks when maximum efficiency is gained. There are also suggestions regarding the time to be spent playing handball, basketball and squash.[5]

Physical exercise not only helps to prevent heart disease. It also prevents further attacks after disease has struck. Findings are that 'active men appear to have two or three times less risk of myocardial infarction and two or three times greater chance of surviving a first heart attack' (than inactive men).[6]

Since energy is used up during physical exercise, exercise leads to loss of weight and should be included in slimming programmes.

Another condition which calls for exercise is diabetes, which is far more prevalent in people who lead sedentary lives than in those who are physically active. It has been found that 'the prevalence of diabetes is very low (0·1 per cent or less) in un-mechanized primitive societies, rising to high levels (up to seven per cent in some cases) in under-exercising industrial communities with extended life span'.[7] Exercise is recommended for established diabetics,[8] and it has been pointed out that better circulation in the muscles during exercise leads to a decrease in blood sugar, thus tending to normalize the metabolic error which constitutes diabetes (although insulin may also be necessary in severe cases).

Autogenic training

Civilized man not only urgently needs bodily activity, but also, definitely, requires relaxation. When you hold yourself correctly in standing, sitting and walking, your posture strikes the right balance between tension and limpness – avoiding, as shown earlier, the two extremes of slumping and of a cramped position. But you must also be trained to relax completely, which is best achieved while lying down in a quiet room in semi-darkness. As is the case with exercises, there are numerous schools of thought. A successful method, which incorporates some of the yoga principles adapted for Western man, was devised by J. H. Schultz. It has proved its success for many years, especially in Germany, and is known as 'Autogenic Training'. It 'improves self-regulatory functions and thus not only enhances a person's overall capacity for psychophysiological adaption but also increases bodily resistance to all kinds of stress'.[9]

If you should undergo this training, changes will be brought about in your body and mind which will affect your muscle-tone, your peripheral blood circulation, your heart-beat, your breathing, and the circulation in your abdomen. You will be taught to become aware of the conditions in these parts of your body and, throughout your training, auto-suggestion, aimed at achieving calmness, will be practised. Thus, as in Natural Therapy, vital functions on which health depends are improved, and the patient takes an active part in the training and is not treated merely as an object of medical science.

In order to reduce outside disturbances, autogenic training is carried out in a quiet, dimly-lit room, with the patient lying down or sitting in a comfortable position. You shut your eyes and are then told to suggest to yourself 'I am calm'. To achieve calmness, you have to learn to bring about the right mood, which must be maintained throughout the subsequent phases of the training. You then start the exercises concerned with the various bodily functions.

As a trainee, you first learn to achieve the sensation of heaviness, which starts in the right arm if you are right-handed, and in the left arm if you are left-handed. Gradually, calmness and heaviness merge into one experience and muscular tension is eliminated. After two to five minutes, you return to your wakeful state through a quick flexion of your elbows; this is followed by taking a deep breath and opening your eyes. Many people feel refreshed after they have been taught to relax their muscles with a feeling of calmness. After you have mastered the sensation of heaviness, you will be introduced to the next phase in which calmness and heaviness are followed by a feeling of warmth, again starting from the right or left arm. The physiological effect is on the blood vessels which become relaxed (they have their own musculature which provides the tonus of the vessel). With the sensation of warmth goes a deepening of the calming effect; feelings of heaviness and warmth fuse into one experience.

From calmness, heaviness and warmth, you proceed to influencing your heart-beat by suggesting to yourself 'my heart is beating calmly'. This experience is particularly valuable for anxious people who suffer from palpitations and from a feeling of oppression.

After having reached awareness of tranquillity through heaviness, warmth and a calm heart-beat, your attention will be concentrated on your breathing: in particular on a gentle up-and-down movement of your chest and abdomen, the movements being associated in your mind with the rhythm of life itself. (Apart from the general relaxing effect, beneficial for people in general, asthmatics in particular can expect benefit from this stage.)

When all these exercises have been perfected, the Therapist will direct your attention to the stomach region and will suggest to you that the nerves around your stomach produce a feeling of warmth. Again, a variety of subjective experiences will coincide with the relaxation of your stomach; the abdominal cavity will feel alive and integrated within the calm flow of life that pervades the rest of your body.

During the last stage of this physiological-psychological training, your concentration will be focused on the forehead. Here, in contrast to the feeling of warmth which has enveloped the rest of your body, you are taught to suggest to yourself 'My forehead is slightly cool'. This pleasant sensation will add to the total experience of relaxation.

It takes from three to four months for a patient to achieve proficiency in the various stages. But with the aid of this training, you can come to terms with the tension of life and can recover from the effects of strain. Many people find that their memory and other mental functions, especially concentration, improve, as does the quality of sleep. (When the various exercises are carried out before going to sleep, the quick flexion of the elbows, the deep breathing and the opening of the eyes should be omitted.)

After you have learned to carry out the various stages of this psychosomatic training, you can be introduced to the 'high stage', which is meditative: you are told to imagine that your eyeballs are turning upwards and inwards and you are asked to imagine a colour which expresses to you a sense of harmony. You have now reached a state of contemplation and you are sinking into yourself. You become sure of your identity and you experience clarity about the meaning of your existence.

Many patients will not achieve the spiritual relaxation of this 'high stage'; some will only become adept at one of the earlier stages; for instance becoming aware of the heaviness and warmth of the body. But whatever stage is reached, autogenic training offers an antidote to the rush and tension of life.

8 Allies to Natural Therapy

Homoeopathy, acupuncture, osteopathy and chiropractic are four auxiliary and independent schools of healing which share with Natural Therapy the common principle of trust in the whole-making integrative power of life. Also, like Natural Therapy, they avoid that gross interference with bodily and mental mechanisms which characterizes conventional medical science, and which can be responsible for many dangerous side-effects, while leaving uncorrected the unhealthy conditions that are largely responsible for human illness. These allies to Natural Therapy will now be discussed; finally, an account will be given of the relaxing and stimulating effects of massage which is another valuable addition to Natural Therapy.

Homoeopathy
Whereas in conventional medicine a drug is chosen for the treatment of a specific disease such as pneumonia or heart failure, the homoeopathic remedy is aimed at the *whole* person, an attitude which is in tune with Natural treatment by diet, hydrotherapy, breathing exercises, and so on. The artificial division of body and mind, adopted by scientific medicine, is avoided by the homoeopathic school, and a total approach is achieved in the following way. Remedies are first given, in appropriate amounts, to healthy people. The homoeopathic doctor notes the effects of the medicines: psychological changes such as irritability and depression, and physical changes such as palpitations, contractions of the stomach, dilatation of blood vessels etc. These objective signs are, however, not the most important features, for what interests the homoeopathic prescriber is the subjective

aspect: how the person who has taken the medicine, the 'prover', experiences the changes. Is the pain in the head relieved by heat or cold, does the patient generally prefer to be warm or cool, does he feel better in the spring or in the winter, what sort of food does he like or dislike? All these and many other personal responses enter into the account which characterizes a particular remedy, the 'drug picture'.

Now, when the prescriber meets a sick person, he will enquire into the finest details of his physico-mental make-up, and will choose a remedy which will match the patient's total condition with the corresponding drug picture. Thus the *whole* patient is related to the healthy 'prover'. Like is cured by like; hence the word homeopathy: 'homoeo' (like), 'pathy' (suffering).

The amount of drug substances in homoeopathic remedies is, as a rule, very small (thus excluding the danger of toxic effects), and the medicines are specially prepared to ensure homogeneous distribution of the material. In acute diseases, doses are given frequently – every half hour in very critical conditions, and evenly two to four hours in less dangerous circumstances. When the organism has responded, the homoeopathic medicine is withdrawn and, in a chronic disease, after the response has begun, no more drug stimulus is applied until the amelioration is complete.

Homoeopathic remedies are derived from the mineral, vegetable and animal kingdom. Let us look at an example of each.

A mineral substance is *natrum muriaticum*, common salt, prepared according to the rule of homoeopathy. This is used for people who have lost weight, who are irritable and reject sympathy, and who tend to suffer from throbbing headaches (in women especially during and after the period). The *natrum muriaticum* patient is constipated, the skin is often inflamed, and the patient feels better in the open air, but not in sea air.

An example of a vegetable remedy is a preparation of *anemone-pulsatilla*. In contrast to the previous picture, here we have a patient who is weepy and craves for sympathy, whose symptoms change frequently, and whose pains shift from one place to another. The patient suffers from digestive upsets after eating rich food and, although the mouth is dry, is not thirsty. In women, the periods are scanty and irregular. Sleep is delayed and restless, a warm room or a close atmosphere is not tolerated, and fresh air is a necessity.

Snake venom, *lachesis*, is one of the remedies derived from the animal kingdom, and is given especially to women who are suspicious, have a vivid imagination and are loquacious. The troubles which occur at the change of life, the irritability and the flushes, are often helped by this remedy. *Lachesis* patients feel worse before the period (which may be irregular during the change), but better when the flow is established. There is a tendency to bleed from small wounds. This drug cures conditions which are similar to those induced by a snake bite.

The number of drugs available is constantly being increased. At present about two thousand are known, but homoeopathy also has its limitations. The Therapist has to keep other measures in readiness if the patient requires them; an urgent operation may have to be performed in the case of a perforated stomach ulcer, a deficiency may have to be made good as is the case in diabetes when insulin must be given, or a weakened heart may need digitalis, and so on. Apart from such urgent needs for scientific medicine, the limitations of homoeopathy lie in its dependence on the possibility of matching the patient's personality with a detailed drug picture. The greater the similarity of the patient's condition to one of the known drug pictures, the better are the chances of helping him.

How does the homoeopathic remedy act? Not through the drug substance as a conventional pharmacological agent. According to the homoeopathic school, the remedy acts through the healing power of Nature, evident in the patient's response. This, of course, accords with the basic tenet of Natural Therapy. Thus the two schools are complementary.[1] Dr Samuel Hahnemann, the founder of homoeopathic medicine, accepted Natural Therapy; he insisted that a patient's mode of living, including his diet, must be corrected before the stimulus of the homoeopathic medicine can be expected to effect a cure.

Having discovered the appropriate homoeopathic medicine, it can be of assistance in the choice of the correct natural stimulus. For instance, responses to heat and cold form essential features in homoeopathic drug pictures. It follows that a patient whose medicine has been worked out to be a remedy suitable for chilly people cannot be expected to respond to cold water treatment. The three examples, given above, *natrum muriaticum*, *anemone*, and *lachesis* are all remedies which fit people who can stand cold temperatures well, but a *natrum muriaticum* patient cannot tolerate sea air, hence the Natural Therapist may advocate as a change of scenery a stay in the country or in the mountains.

In the homoeopathic drug picture we may find a combination of afflictions of the skin, such as eczema, and in the chest, such as asthma. The remedy, amorphous carbon, will tend to be helpful for both the conditions, thus restoring the disturbed equilibrium which the Natural Therapist restores by his use of natural stimuli.

Temporary aggravations are expected by both the Natural Therapy and the homoeopathic schools. The possible beneficial 'cleansing' effect of an attack of diarrhoea was mentioned earlier (page 21), and under homoeopathic treatment such healing responses are often brought about soon after a remedy has been given. Such a reaction confirms that the drug was chosen correctly.

Homoeopathic and conventional medicine meet in the prevention of specific infections, although they differ on dosage and methods of application. The conventional school carries out immunization against such infectious illnesses as diphtheria, whooping cough and influenza, and particular toxins are injected into the patient in order to stimulate the formation of antibodies and to prevent an attack of the disease. The homoeopathic school uses dilutions of the poison of these infections in order either to prevent an attack or to help the patient to recover from the after-effects of one.

As regards the difference in dosage, the small or infinitesimal dose is not an essential feature of homoeopathic medicine; homoeopathy's fundamental tenet is the matching of the remedy with the patient. It is, however, true that many homoeopathic physicians prescribe 'potencies' which lie outside the molecular limit; this means that, for instance, a 30. potency of sulphur does not contain any sulphur. The homoeopath, however, claims that it contains some energy derived from the original sulphur which has now entered the medium in which the sulphur was diluted (for instance, spirit or sugar), and which could manifest itself through specific sulphur radiations.

All this is speculation. The homoeopath points out that the efficacy of his preparations, including the high potencies has been proved empirically over more than 150 years. And, although some of these 'potencies' do not contain any of the material from which they were derived, it does not follow that they are ineffective. Let us remember that modern physicists do not hold that, ultimately, the universe consists of matter. From a philosophical point of view it must be pointed out that matter, molecules and energy are concepts created by the scientist's mind and are not part of the reality of Nature. The world, apart from the knowing mind, is inscrutable.[2,3]

Acupuncture

By dropping a few granules of sugar, impregnated with a specially diluted remedy on a patient's tongue, the homoeopath sets nature's vitalizing power into motion. Similarly, by touching certain points on a patient's skin with a fine needle, the acupuncturist mobilizes the same force.

Acupuncture has been practised in China for thousands of years, and the Chinese explain its efficacy in a metaphysical way. They maintain that the unity of life embodies a negative principle, Yin, and a positive principle Yang. An assumption of the existence of these two forces is not confined to the field of biology, but pervades the whole of Chinese life and is found in art, literature and philosophy. The interplay of Yin and Yang is traced as a rhythmical movement throughout the universe, which is explained in this polar manner; any disturbance of the relationship between the two poles constitutes disharmony, which in medicine stands for disease.

The acupuncturist defines channels through which the life energy flows: they are the 'meridians' which follow a well-defined course on the body surface. By inserting fine needles into these 'meridians' he claims that the disturbed balance can be restored and a cure brought about. The Natural Therapist steeped in Western thought, cannot accept the dualistic metaphysical conception but he can accept the concept of harmony standing for health and wholeness. He might explain the effects of the pricking of the skin in terms of a reflex. The skin is richly supplied with nerves, and these are connected with the spinal cord, with the brain, and, indirectly, with all the organs in the body.[4] For instance, tension of the muscles in the back, distorting the spine and thus affecting the rest of the body, can be relieved by acupuncture. In this way, great help can be given to the vast number of people who suffer from backache. Such patients are not only physically tense, they also suffer from emotional tension, and by the use of acupuncture both forms of tension may be removed.[5]

The acupuncturist accepts relationships between the skin and the internal organs in a way which differs from the teachings of the medical schools. For instance, he considers that a disturbed liver causes migraine, allergic conditions, gout, poor eyesight, and general tiredness and weakness. He asserts that by stimulating the liver through the skin, all these conditions can be cured. From the point of view of Natural Therapy, the liver is of importance as the large detoxicating organ; thus, acupuncture, directed to the liver meridian, may assist the cleansing efforts which are encouraged during a fast or an eliminative diet. Since the days of the ancient Greeks, the liver, the producer of the gall, has been associated with a 'choleric' temperament. A Natural Therapist is aware of the emotional effects of a toxic physical condition. Similarly, the Chinese acupuncturist refers to the liver as 'the sect of the Unconscious'; thus, by treating the liver, he is convinced that he treats the mind.[6]

Some modern Western medical acupuncturists also claim to influence the mind directly. Dr Paul Renard, for instance, has related acupuncture to the tenets of the various schools of psychological medicine, and, at the same time, to the drug pictures of certain homoeopathic remedies.[7] We have seen that homoeopathy also considers the patient as a psychosomatic unit, and the relationship between acupuncture and homoeopathy is accepted by other French acupuncturists besides Renard.

Following Renard, we may assume that the mind is 'accessible' to the acupuncturist, as he has proved that he can deeply influence the nervous system, that he can abolish the sensation of pain to such a degree that major operations can be carried out without any ordinary anaesthetic. A modification of brain activity may well amount to a change in mental activity.

The Chinese acupuncturist pays great attention to the pulse and is trained to feel fourteen different pulses above the wrist. In this way, he judges the conditions of the organs throughout the body.

Dr Otto Bergsmann, working with Dr J. Bischko at the Vienna Institute for the Study of Acupuncture (Das Ludwig-Boltzmann Institut für Akupunktur), has related certain points situated on the skin to certain pathological processes in the lungs. These authors have explained the effect of acupuncture in terms of a *regulation* of bodily activities, and they have developed new methods which are suitable for this type of research.[8] This is an example of integrating the knowledge gained by Chinese workers into the field of scientific medicine. As we have seen, a regulative force is postulated also by homoeopathy and by Natural Therapy; it is a manifestation of nature's vital force. It is also a fundamental concept in the systems of osteopathy and chiro-practic, further allies of Natural Therapy.

Osteopathy

The manipulations which are used in conjunction with the methods of Natural Therapy belong to the special field of *osteopathy* and *chiropractic*. The principles of osteopathy have been interpreted within the conceptual framework of modern sciences,[9] and the effects of this mechanical treatment can be understood in terms of cybernetics, the science which is concerned with controls and communications within a system. It is thought that equilibrium is achieved by 'negative feedback': part of the output of surplus energy is diverted in order to achieve a balance. In the living organism, communications between different parts occur through reflex activity, and disturbances in this channel can be the result of mechanical faults such as sprains, obstructions of lymph and blood vessels, and immobilization of joints. Any disturbance in the bodily structure which is apt to lead to a disturbance of function is called an *osteopathic lesion*, and since it affects muscles and bones, it is 'muscoskeletal'. The disturbance may consist of a restriction of mobility within a section of the spine, interfering with the reflexes that extend from the spinal column to other parts of the body, including the internal organs. The lesion interrupts the feedback and a correction by the osteopath restores normal functioning of the dynamic pattern. Not only does the mechanical fault cause biochemical disturbances in the tissues, a biochemical disturbance can itself cause mechanical malfunctioning. Such biochemical faults may result from a disturbed function of a nerve and may be amenable to manipulations of the spine. Thus, the osteopath claims that he can release spasm in the intestines, regulate the heart-beat and correct abnormal circulation in different parts of the body.

Two types of osteopathic lesion are distinguished: the primary lesion resulting from an abnormal stimulus originating in the spine which has caused some alteration within the body, and the secondary osteopathic lesion which has developed as the outcome of some visceral irritation or other abnormal functioning within the organism. The result is a faulty posture which causes pain and tenderness in the affected areas. The body responds to the irritation with alteration in elasticity, in fluid content, in texture, in temperature, in colour, in vascular supply and in abnormal electrical conditions. Experiments on animals are said to have confirmed the theory of the osteopathic lesion and its physiological consequences, and further evidence has been collected through examining the changes in the muscles and nerves of human beings.

The osteopath uses technical manoeuvres which affect the various parts of the body: lymphatic drainage through special massage, movements of the chest wall which affect the heart and the blood vessels inside the chest, and manipulation of joints with special reference to the vertebral column. It is also claimed that manipulative therapy 'can play a major role' in the treatment of ulcers in the stomach and duodenum. In case of inflammation in the kidneys, the correction of osteopathic lesions is said to improve the circulation and thus assist in the healing. Manipulative osteopathic treatment to the lower part of the spine is employed for the relief of bladder troubles, and allergic diseases are said to respond to manipulations of the spine, as such manipulations reduce the exaggerated sensitivity which is the cause of the condition. Bronchial asthma is one of the allergic conditions for which an osteopathic technique has been devised.[10]

While employing specific techniques, osteopathic treatment relies on the integration of the whole body; in this respect osteopaths accept the fundamental conception of Natural Therapy. They also admit limitations to their system of healing, and accept the need for the conventional methods of scientific medicine in some conditions.

Chiropractic

The osteopath, as we have seen, pays special, although not exclusive, attention to the spinal column. The chiropractor concentrates his treatment entirely on the vertebrae. Chiropractic is a system which adjusts by hand the alignments of the vertebrae, correcting faulty positions and restoring normal mobility. The correction is carried out by thrusts while the patient lies on a table which is sprung. Parnell Bradbury claims to have integrated osteopathy and chiropractic in his system of 'spinology' – explained in his book *The Mechanics of Healing*. As the name 'spinology' indicates, attention is confined to the spine. In a foreword, Dr Dudley Tee has confirmed that beneficial responses in patients were accompanied by changes in the blood sugar level and by other alterations within the body.[11]

Massage
Massage can either be given to the patient by a professional person or the patient can be taught to massage himself.

Professional massage
Spinal manipulations are often combined with massage which is chiefly applied to the large muscles situated on either side of the spine. The beneficial effects of acupuncture are also improved if the muscular relaxation which is achieved by the insertion of the fine needles is followed by firm rubbing.

Acupuncture effects can, in fact, be achieved by massage of the points into which the acupuncturist inserts his needles, these areas being 'trigger points', sensitive areas from which nervous impulses travel to other parts of the body. Thus massage not only relieves local conditions such as sprains, congestion and tension, but also influences parts of the body which are connected by reflexes with the area which is massaged. A general massage provides relaxation and is of physical and psychological benefit. Mrs Elisabeth Dicke has discovered a further important use. Her technique consists in pushing the skin with the third and fourth fingers against underlying tissues such as bone, tendons and muscles. The resulting pull constitutes a stimulus which affects the nervous system, the blood and lymph, and the cells situated under the skin which are concerned with drainage of waste products deposited in the tissues. Dicke found that areas which had become hardened could become soft again, and that remarkable relief could be given to patients suffering from a disturbance of circulation. Her connective tissue massage always starts at the base of the spine and extends upwards.[12]

Self-massage
Apart from receiving treatment from a trained person, those who adopt natural methods may apply massage to their own bodies.

Techniques for the abdomen, the legs, and the tonsillar region will now be described and, finally, it will be suggested how the whole body can benefit from vigorous brushing or towelling.

Self-massage of abdomen

This form of massage aims at stimulating the bowels and is therefore helpful in constipation and flatulence. (It should not be used in cases of inflammation, which are often characterized by pain.) The patient lies on the back with the knees flexed. The right hand pressed against the right lower part of the abdomen while the left hand, lying on top of the right hand, increases the pressure. Now, both hands move upwards towards the ribs, then across the stomach to the left side, and then downwards. This whole movement is performed while breathing out. The breath is taken in while the hands resume their starting position on the right side. The movements are repeated fifteen to twenty times.

Another type of abdominal self-massage consists in using the fingers of the right hand as a hammer which, through movements of the wrists, taps against the various parts of the abdomen. The tapping should be very gentle in the upper part where the stomach is situated and should not be applied to the part in the centre, where the bladder lies. The tapping takes place while breathing out, and follows the same route as the abdominal massage described earlier.

Abdominal self-massage can be carried out very effectively without using the hands, by a jerking movement of the abdominal muscles. The position is the same as when self-massage of the abdomen is given. The abdomen is drawn in and jerked out. This in-and-out movement is repeated fifteen to twenty times. The back does not move and is not raised. The breathing rhythm is not disturbed; inspiration takes place during two to four of the flicker movements, expiration during four to six. It is important that the quick movements of the diaphragm do not interfere with proper breathing. If carried out correctly, this form of self-massage is very beneficial for those conditions which respond to ordinary abdominal self-massage. (The same precautions obtain with regard to inflammatory diseases.)

Self-massage of legs

The person lies on the back and bends the right leg so that the right foot can be grasped with both hands. Both hands then begin the self-massage from the toes, with stroking movements which extend upwards beyond the knee. These movements are repeated about five times and then the calf is shaken vigorously with both hands, starting from the heel and going up to the knee. The calf muscles are further relaxed through hacking movements, using the edge of the fifth finger and the adjacent part of the hand, again starting from the heel. Now the muscles of the thigh are firmly stroked with both hands in an upward direction, and then shaken. Next, hacking movements are applied to the thigh in the same manner as to the calf. Several large stroking movements from the toes to the hips complete the massage, which is then repeated on the left leg. The self-massage aids the circulation in the legs and is also used in cases of cramps. It should not be used where there is inflammation, or in cases of varicose veins since clots situated in the veins could be dislodged and cause serious disturbances in other parts of the circulatory system.

Self-massage of tonsils

The tonsils and the surrounding tissues belong to the lymphatic system; this is concerned with the mobilization of defences against invading micro-organisms. Natural Therapists assume that the tonsils are related to various glands within the body, to the organs concerned with digestion of food, and to the nervous system – especially to certain parts of the brain. Thus, tonsillar massage has far-reaching stimulating effects. It also aids the clearing of material which has accumulated in the tonsillar crypts, and it can be helpful in cases of catarrh in the upper part of the throat. The massage is carried out with the index finger. If the tonsils are inflamed, the treatment should not be applied, as it could lead to an aggravation of the inflammation which might affect other parts of the body, especially the kidneys. Tonsillar massage can be made more effective by means of suction applied through a glass tube and operated by means of a rubber bulb.

Whole-body brushing or rough towelling
Vigorous brushing or rough towelling can stimulate the skin and indirectly, the whole body. The treatment starts from the right arm and is directed towards the heart. Next, the left arm is treated, followed by the front of the body, and then the back. Finally, the feet and legs are rubbed.

9 Twelve case histories

Natural Therapy and its auxiliary methods will now be illustrated by quoting twelve cases. Although each has been identified with the name of an illness, it should be remembered that treatment, which is based on the idea of wholeness, is not so much given for the specific disease as for the patient who suffers from it. In each case, the question asked was: in what respect has the patient, in his mode of living, neglected the principles on which health (i.e. wholeness) depends? In trying to restore him to health (wholeness), the Therapist had to assess what response to the natural methods could be expected.

Case 1: Recurrent boils
A man of 42 had been plagued with boils for seven years. They had started near his left ear but had then affected the sweat glands in his armpits. He had received enormous amounts of penicillin, also X-ray treatment, and an incision had been made in his left axilla. Finally, a major operation by a plastic surgeon – the removal of a large part of the affected skin – had been advised.

The Natural Therapist enquired into the patient's diet – something which had never been done before. It transpired that this man was in the habit of taking ten cups of tea per day, putting four teaspoonsful of sugar into each. In addition, he drank coffee sweetened with sugar, enjoyed carbohydrates such as jam, puddings and sweet biscuits, and smoked 40 to 60 cigarettes a day.

The treatment consisted in the elimination of all sugar, coffee and tea, and the man was told that he must stop smoking. He was put on a diet: mostly raw fruit and raw vegetables with

cottage cheese and yoghurt as protein. He also received a
homoeopathic medicine, Hepar Sulphuris, which is helpful in
cases of boils.

The patient made excellent progress. In the first two weeks his
weight dropped from 12 stone 2 lb (77·2 kg) to 11 stone 10 lb
(74·5 kg). He felt better in himself and the inflammation in his
armpits was much reduced. He still craved for cigarettes, however, and smoked about three per day. The man's diet was now
increased by three eggs a week, two Ryvita biscuits per day, and
ordinary cheese.

Four weeks after the start of the treatment, his weight had
become steady, and the boils were small (whereas before there
had been large collections of pus). In order to increase his protein
intake, nuts were added to the diet. The patient was by now
convinced that the new regime was beneficial, and his full
co-operation was won. Eight months after the start of the treatment he was allowed meat, fish and cooked vegetables in addition
to his original diet. The inflammation in his armpits decreased,
so that after one year no more boils appeared. Four and a half
years after his first consultation with the Natural Therapist, his
local doctor reported that there had not been any recurrence of
boils.

The Natural Therapist treated this patient's disease by
eliminating harmful habits and recommending a diet which
consisted largely of uncooked vegetables and fruit. Dairy
produce was introduced from the beginning and later, meat and
fish. Thus the body recovered its powers to deal with the germs
which are present on every skin but which, in this case, had
caused serious trouble.

Case 2: Ulcerative colitis and recurrent virus infection of the skin
A man aged 29 had suffered in his childhood from frequent
attacks of influenza, bronchitis, and from a prolonged fever
which had presumably been caused by a virus. At the age of 19,
he started having attacks of diarrhoea. At the age of 23, there
was blood in his stools and the diagnosis of ulcerative colitis was
made. With the diarrhoea he had bouts of fever which weakened

him considerably and he also suffered abdominal pain. At the age of 28, he had his first attack of herpes simplex, a virus infection of the skin, which recurred frequently and was each time accompanied by looseness of his bowels, loss of appetite and general malaise.

Homoeopathic treatment was started when he was 29, and the remedy, *pyrogen*, which is prepared from septic material, precipitated an attack of diarrhoea accompanied by fever, but then led to recovery from his bowel trouble. Other homoeopathic medicines, such as *cinchona* (Peruvian bark), were also helpful, but his herpes simplex continued to trouble him, causing considerable weakness. At the age of 33, he consulted a Natural Therapist, and in view of his long history, his determination to achieve better health, and his youth, a strict dietetic regime was suggested:

Breakfast
2 grated apples + 2 tablespoonsful of oats soaked in 4 tablespoonsful of water overnight + 1 carton of yoghurt + 1 dessertspoonful of Froment. Apple juice, herb tea.

Lunch
Raw salad without salt and vinegar, oil, lemon juice, Ryvita biscuit, vegetarian margarine, cottage cheese.

Tea-time
Apple juice.

Supper
Another raw salad with fruit, potato in jacket, yoghurt.

Water treatment was also prescribed: a cold sponge of the whole body, morning and night. Later he increased his vitality by carrying out Dr Kenneth Cooper's 'aerobics'. He also received further homoeopathic medicines from time to time.

The patient felt the impact of this frugal way of living and was frightened by the response from his friends who warned him that he would lose strength. When visiting them, he felt that, by rejecting their food, he had rejected them. But, gradually, the patient and his friends got used to the situation, and he so much liked the food that he had no wish to return to his former diet. After three weeks, cooked vegetables were added in the form of 'Vecon', a vegetable powder, to be dissolved in hot water. The soup was thickened and made more nourishing by the addition of unpolished rice.

Under Natural Therapy, the patient experienced immediate relief from an irritation of the skin which had worried him considerably and which had seriously interfered with his sleep. This symptom was interpreted as an expression of his toxic state. The first ten days were difficult; for his body had not learnt to assimilate the food and he felt rather hungry. Then a reaction set in: he suffered from headache, felt very weak, perspired heavily, felt thirsty but not hungry. This was a crisis which was a turning point in his illness. After that, his general condition improved, his sense of taste and of smell improved considerably, he felt less tense, calmer and more energetic, and was looking forward to his work. His bowels recovered except for a short bout of diarrhoea. His attacks of herpes became much milder, and no longer depressed and exhausted him. Natural Therapy had raised his resistance.

This man's case is instructive because, although he had made progress after homoeopathic treatment, he gained a greater measure of health after adopting a Natural Therapy regime.

Case 3: Osteo-arthritis

A woman of sixty-one, weighing 12 stone 6 lb (79 kg) complained that during the past fifteen months she had suffered from pain in her knees which the doctor had diagnosed as osteo-arthritis. She had been ordered tablets for the pain, but they had not given her much relief.

An inquiry into her diet revealed that she ate wholemeal bread, marmalade, Ryvita, cheese, eggs, fruit, meat, fish and yoghurt, and that she drank tea and decaffeinated coffee. She was asked to give up bread, was put on a lacto-vegetarian diet, and was encouraged to sponge her whole body with cold water, morning and night. After three weeks, she had lost seven pounds

(3 kg) and her knee was more comfortable. The knee improved further, she lost another five pounds (2·25 kg) and was able to walk with comfort four and a half months after she had started treatment.

This patient was told that she had to be careful not to gain weight. The treatment was not drastic, but the change in her mode of living proved sufficient to bring about marked improvement.

Case 4: Varicose ulcers

A woman aged 49 and weighing 13 stone 7 lb (85·8 kg), complained of ulcers on her legs. They had first appeared when she was only 12 years old. They had scarred over and for the next 25 years remained healed. When she was 37, she developed an ulcer on her left leg. She attended a Natural Therapist, who prescribed a lacto-vegetarian diet, on which she lost five pounds (2·25 kg). The leg was bandaged to support the venous circulation, homoeopathic medicines were prescribed, and the ulcer gradually diminished in size, healing after one year and nine months.

Eight years later two large ulcers appeared, exuding foul pus. It was decided to admit her to hospital, and to put her on a fast. Tests were carried out to make sure that her heart was fit and that there were no deficiencies in her blood. For twelve days she had only water to drink and was given some vitamins; during this period she lost 21 pounds (9·5 kg) and the ulcers healed. The case was followed up. Two years after the fast, she reported that every second week she had fasted every other day for 24 hours and had thus succeeded in keeping her weight down to a level two stone (12·7 kg) less than it had been before the fast. There was no recurrence of ulceration and she was fit.

Case 5: Cirrhosis of the liver

A middle-aged woman developed jaundice, was admitted to hospital, and diagnosis of cirrhosis of the liver was made. She stayed in hospital for nine weeks and was given cortisone for the following two years. As this drug upset her severely, she refused to take any more. The next year, she put herself on a grape diet for four weeks, eating only several pounds of grapes per day. While on grapes, she felt well and lost the discomfort in her abdomen which had disturbed her before. Her discomfort recurred, however, when she went back to ordinary food.

Two years later she repeated the grape cure on her own, eating four to five pounds (approximately 2 kg) of grapes per day for another four weeks. Again her discomfort disappeared and she felt well, while she lost 21 lbs (9·5 kg) in weight. She then went back to a conventional diet.

As she felt ill again, she consulted a Natural Therapist. She was given a diet which consisted of Weetabix, milk, and orange juice for breakfast; vegetable soup, wholemeal bread and cheese for lunch; and a salad with cheese, occasional eggs, baked potato and some milk for supper. In addition, she received a homoeopathic medicine, made from the Water Ash. (This remedy is suitable for patients with liver and digestive upsets, and thus suited the patient's condition.) Under this dietetic and homoeopathic treatment, the patient made rapid progress, lost her discomfort, and gained four pounds (1·8 kg) in one month,

Conventional medicine has no special treatment for cirrhosis of the liver and patients are not given a special diet although they are advised to avoid alcohol. In this case, a small piece of liver tissue (biopsy) had been examined and the diagnosis had been confirmed. The patient had been told that her condition was likely to improve, but this did not occur until Natural Therapy, which included the use of the appropriate homoeopathic remedy, was instituted.

Case 6: A catarrhal child
A little girl, aged two, was brought to a Natural Therapist with a history of frequent colds, constant thick yellow nasal discharge, and frequent attacks of ear-ache. She was put on a diet consisting of muesli, lemon juice and honey for breakfast; cheese salad and fruit for lunch; and meat or fish, cooked vegetables, potatoes in their skins, and fruit for supper.

When she was seen about three years later, the mother reported that there had been no more colds nor any nasal discharge while she was on the diet, but that she had recently started eating school lunches and had also deviated from her diet when invited to other children's homes where white bread and cakes were provided. The catarrh in her nose had returned and blocked her nostrils, tending to make her breathe through her mouth.

The Natural Therapist gave a certificate to enable the child to take a packed salad lunch to school, and also instructed the mother to encourage the child to breathe through her nose, to remind her of it during the day and, if possible, to close her mouth with a firm elastic strap under the chin at night. In addition, she received a homoeopathic medicine, *Silica 30*.

This case illustrates a common problem. Children are subjected to operations on their tonsils and adenoids and are given antibodies for coughs and ear-ache, when the correct treatment is in fact a reform of their diet, a cutting out of white flour, eaten as pastry and white bread, and of sugar, consumed in sweets. School lunches and the conventional teas offered to children at home, especially at parties, are a potent factor in keeping the catarrhal condition going, and this case shows how difficult it is for a child to remain a member of his or her group and still to continue on a healthy diet.

Case 7: Rheumatoid arthritis

A woman aged 38 was taken ill with swellings of many joints and a fever. She was diagnosed as a case of acute rheumatoid arthritis, lost 21 lbs (9·5 kg) in weight, and became very weak and anaemic. She was discharged from a hospital where she had not made any progress, and was first seen by a Natural Therapist two years after the onset of the illness. He found that the joints in her arms and legs were swollen and painful. The skin on her face was inflamed, there were cracks at the corners of her mouth, scaling on her scalp and her nails were brittle. She coughed and brought up some yellow phlegm. She was constipated. She had ceased to menstruate. An inquiry into her diet showed that it had been conventional: she had bacon and eggs, bread, butter and milk for breakfast; vegetables, meat, and grilled tomatoes for lunch;

sometimes fish, tomatoes, bread, butter, milk and egg for tea;
and bread and milk for supper.

The Natural Therapist modified her diet by reducing the meat
to twice a week, ordering yoghurt as the main form of protein,
introducing more raw vegetables, but also allowing some cooked
vegetables, and adding oats and blackcurrant puree as an
additional source of vitamin C. After the first week, he reduced
the meat to once a week and then cut it out completely. For
further protein, she took soya preparations and nut cream, and
was also allowed brown unpolished rice.

Her knees had become fixed in a flexed state. In order to
straighten them, a pulley was fixed to the end of her bed and
weights were attached. To help the functions of her skin, she was
sponged all over with lukewarm water three times a day. She was
given a homoeopathic medicine which helps patients with
arthritis – a dilution of the poison oak.

Her bowels became regular, her knees straight and her fever
subsided, but her skin remained inflamed and itchy. Two further
homoeopathic remedies helped her in this respect – petroleum
and the spurge olive. Her stools were cultured to investigate her
bowel flora, and the next homoeopathic remedy consisted of a
dilution of the prevalent organisms: bacillus proteus. This last
prescription caused some aggravation in the pain of her joints
but she soon felt better, and thus the reaction was beneficial.
Her joints improved and her cough lessened.

This treatment had commenced in May of one year and by the
January of the next her menstrual period returned, another sign
of a general recovery. By February of that year, her knees had
become straight, she could move them normally and she started
to walk again. By April her chest was clear. In June her stools
became loose and she reported that the pain in her joints was
relieved by passing the motion. Thus, no attempt was made to
control the diarrhoea, as it was obviously helping in the healing
process. By April of the following year, the patient was sleeping
better, she could walk for forty-five minutes, and had gained two
stone (12·7 kg) in weight, and her skin was practically normal.
She received several further homoeopathic medicines, amongst

them a preparation made from the cuttle fish, which improved her emotional state.

The patient kept in touch with her Therapist for the next 39 years. Her arthritis never caused her any marked disability. She led an active life, got married and was able to look after a big house. She never deviated from her lacto-vegetarian diet.

This case demonstrates the beneficial effects of Natural Therapy in a patient crippled with rheumatoid arthritis. As was pointed out in the first chapter, this condition is very common and the sufferers are mostly treated with drugs to relieve their pain. In contrast to such purely symptomatic palliative treatment, Natural Therapy gets to the root of the trouble and restores health by stimulating the defences of the body. The patient's progress showed how the skin, the linings of the bronchial tubes and the micro-organisms in the bowels were all involved, and how their condition was improved by the natural methods. The looseness of the bowel was interpreted as a healing effort to eliminate toxic material. The patient's attitude was of vital importance. By adopting Natural Therapy as her new way of life, she obtained lasting benefit.

Case 8: Heart failure

A man of 67 was admitted to hospital with a heart attack (occlusion of one of the blood vessels within the heart muscle). He was discharged after three weeks, suffering from breathlessness and swollen ankles, signs of heart failure.

He then consulted a Natural Therapist, who found that his breakfast consisted of four cups of tea with milk and sugar, his lunch of white bread sandwiches with cheese, tomatoes and lettuce, and his supper of meat or fish with vegetables. This diet was drastically changed. For the first two weeks he was allowed only raw vegetables, Weetabix, yoghurt and cheese. He was told to sponge his whole body with cold water, and he received a homoeopathic medicine, sulphur, which suited his constitution.

There was an immediate improvement and he found he could walk without getting breathless. After one month he was allowed some cooked vegetables and an occasional egg. After two months, he reported that he could walk for two and a half miles without getting breathless or tired. His weight had dropped from 12 stone (75·5 kg) to 10 stone 2 lb (64·5 kg), and had now become almost stationary. Further foods – honey, Ryvita biscuits, wholemeal bread, some milk, and meat three times a week – were added two weeks later.

This case demonstrates that Natural Therapy can be of great benefit in cases of heart failure and that after an initial strict regime, the patient can be allowed a fairly full diet, provided white flour and sugar are excluded.

Case 9: Advanced nephritis

A young man aged 24 was taken ill with the signs of an inflamma-tion of his kidneys (nephritis). He had albumen in his urine and evidence of kidney disease in his blood. He was treated by an eminent specialist in kidney diseases. The illness advanced to a chronic state and the patient's father was informed that chances of a cure were minimal. The only conventional treatment consisted of prolonged rest in bed and avoidance of salt in the diet, but this regime did not make any difference to the patient's condition.

He had eaten the usual type of food – meat, fish, white bread – and had drunk tea and coffee. As he was determined to try Natural Therapy, he put himself on a stricter diet consisting of fruit and orange juice for breakfast, brown bread sandwiches with egg, cheese and marmite for lunch, orange juice at tea-time, and meat, fish, eggs, macaroni, vegetables, pastry and fruit for supper.

He began treatment with a Natural Therapist two months later, when he was given a very strict diet: muesli and raw vegetables only. He was encouraged to take air and sun baths and was instructed in breathing exercises. He also received a homoeopathic medicine, *Kali Arsenicosum*, which benefits sufferers from nephritis. There was a quick response to the combined Natural and homoeopathic treatments; he felt better in himself. Then his stools became loose and offensive; this was interpreted as an effort on the part of his body to eliminate toxic material, and no attempt was made to stop the diarrhoea.

After three months, there was some objective improvement; the excretion of albumen in his urine had diminished. Another homoeopathic medicine, also helpful in kidney diseases, *Kali Iodatum*, was prescribed. The looseness of the bowels persisted for some time, while the general condition improved.

After seven months on natural treatment, he was still feeling rather tense. Autogenic training was begun; the patient learned to relax and to experience heaviness, warmth, calm heart action, calm breathing, and warmth in the nerve centre of the abdomen. Eleven months after the start of the treatment, his weight had increased from 8 stone 5½ lb (53·5 kg) – at the beginning of the treatment – to 9 stone 1 lb (57·5 kg). At that time, some cream cheese and wholemeal bread were added to the diet. Eight months later he introduced cooked vegetables and yoghurt as well as eggs and nuts into his diet, and six months later there was no longer any albumen in his urine.

This patient remained on a lacto-vegetarian diet and had at least one raw salad meal every day. He had regular checkups for his kidney trouble and the last thorough examination was carried out when he was 45, 21 years from the start of his Natural Therapy treatment. He was assured that he was completely cured.

A case of advanced inflammation of the kidneys, for which there was no treatment in conventional scientific medicine, was cured by Natural Therapy including homoeopathy and autogenic training. The patient's excellent cooperation made the prolonged strict treatment possible.

Case 10: Acne vulgaris

The acne started in this girl's case at the age of twelve when her menstrual periods commenced. Ointments and exposure to artificial ultra-violet light and even to X-rays were tried. When she was nineteen, she attended the skin department of the Royal London Homoeopathic Hospital. By then her face was severely disfigured by redness, pustules, large bags of pus and thick scar formation. There were also pustules on her chest and back. She received homoeopathic medicines, a high dilution of the common salt (*natrum muriaticum*) and of sulphur. There was some improvement, but as she had not changed her eating habits, the improvement did not last. For the next two and a half years, she took an antibiotic which kept her condition under control. Then she had to stop the drug, as the side-effects had become too disturbing.

The turning point in this case was reached when the girl's diet was changed. She had been consuming too much carbohydrates: her breakfast had consisted of Bran Flakes and coffee, her lunch of biscuits and Energen bread, her evening meal of meat, vegetables and a sweet. The Natural Therapist decided that a strict regime was necessary and that the emphasis should lie on raw fruit and raw vegetables. Breakfast was altered to a mixture of oats, apples, froment and yoghurt, a modification of the muesli; lunch and the evening meal consisted of raw salad, cottage cheese and a potato in its skin or a piece of Ryvita. As it was winter, vegetable soup was allowed to keep her warm, but tea and coffee were excluded. This strict diet was kept up for six weeks, when other items were introduced, but pastry, chocolate and fried foods were eaten only seldom. Even after twelve years, raw vegetable and cooked vegetables were still important items in her diet. A number of homoeopathic medicines were prescribed: *kali bromatum*, which has a close relationship to acne pustules; a mixture of sulphur, silica and vegetable charcoal which is beneficial in septic conditions in general, and sulphur in a high dilution which has a deep constitutional effect.

The result of this combined natural and homoeopathic treatment was highly satisfactory: the bags of pus and pustules went and the skin assumed a normal texture. There was also a marked improvement in the patient's general health: she lost previous pains in her head and back and also an unpleasant taste, a sign of elimination of toxins through the mouth.

This case demonstrates the beneficial effects of a Natural

Therapy diet on a chronic inflammatory condition of the skin.
By restricting the intake of carbohydrates and fats, the secretion
of the fatty substance (sebum) is reduced and the skin thus
becomes less greasy and less inflamed. It should be noted that the
patient wholly recovered.

Case 11: Multiple sclerosis

A woman aged 30 developed typical signs of multiple sclerosis:
transient difficulty of vision, tenderness, numbness, stiffness and
heaviness of her legs with progressive weakness which made
walking difficult. A specialist was consulted who found the power
of her right leg had been diminished by 80 to 90 per cent, of her
left leg by 50 per cent. Within a few days, the power in the left leg
decreased further.

She consulted a Natural Therapist who prescribed a drastic
change from her conventional diet. He followed the instructions
given by the German physician, Dr Evers, who had found that
sprouting wheat and rye benefited patients suffering from
multiple sclerosis. The value of sprouting grains has already been
stressed. As we saw, they are extremely rich in various vitamins
and they contain first-class proteins. The patient followed the
instructions for sprouting and keeping the grains clean (see
page 53). In addition she was allowed every day two pints of
milk, one raw egg and raw grated root vegetables. She also
received a homoeopathic remedy, prepared from an Indian
Vetch.

There was an immediate improvement: the strength of her legs
increased and the spasm lessened. Hot compresses were applied
to relax the stiff muscles. Within two months, the patient had a fair
degree of mobility and was able to co-ordinate her movements.
As her gait was still uncertain, however, she was put in touch
with a teacher of the Matthias Alexander system (see page 86).
Already, in the first lesson, the patient's sense of balance was
restored. She continued the exercises for a while and derived
further benefit from them.

After two months of treatment, her diet was increased: she
added wholemeal bread and a full salad (including leaf

vegetables), but she kept off tea and coffee for a whole year, and off alcohol for two years.

After four months on the regime she was practically well. There was only some slight unsteadiness of her hands, and she felt ready to look for a job again. After a further four months, she complained of tiredness and jerking of one leg. Two homoeopathic medicines, prepared from lead and the poison nut (*nux vomica*), brought relief. She was also given breathing exercises which she continued. Her last consultation was 15 months from the beginning of the treatment. Apart from some difficulty in falling asleep and slight twitching of her legs, she had no complaints. She received a high potency of the poison hemlock.

She got married and had two children. 20 years after she had started the treatment, she reported that she was still following a lacto-vegetarian diet. She always took wholemeal bread. Her health was excellent and she had not suffered any recurrence of her symptoms. At the age of 50 she took up tennis!

Multiple sclerosis is a disease which fluctuates. In this case the recovery followed immediately upon the commencement of a comprehensive treatment on natural lines, including diet, water treatment, massage, exercises and homoeopathic medicine. The excellent permanent cure must be attributed to Natural Therapy which the patient continued, having adopted its principles as a way of living.

Case 12: Acute sinusitis

A woman aged 43 consulted a Natural Therapist on account of an attack of acute nasal sinusitis. She had been ill for three days, and an antibiotic had given little relief. She had a slight temperature, her nose felt stuffy, and she had a severe headache.

She was put on a strict diet consisting of fruit, yoghurt, raw salad and cottage cheese. She received an acupuncture treatment which immediately freed her nasal passage and relieved her headache. In addition she was given a homoeopathic medicine, made from slaked lime. She recovered, but was advised to continue with the strict diet for two weeks, and then to add some cooked food.

This case has been quoted to illustrate the handling of an acute illness by Natural Therapy. If the fever is high, fasting on water and fruit juices is prescribed, and cold compresses around the waist are applied in order to encourage the elimination of toxins through the skin. Appropriate homoeopathic medicines are also used. In less acute cases, such as this one, raw vegetables and fruit with yoghurt constitute a suitable diet.

Notes

1 The rising tide of illness

1 Dunlop, Sir Derrick. 'Use and Abuse of Drugs', *British Medical Journal* 21 August 1965

2 Barr, D. P. 'Hazards of Modern Diagnosis and Therapy – The Price we Pay', *Journal of the American Medical Association* 159 1452, 1955; quoted in Laurence, D. R. *Clinical Pharmacology* Churchill Livingstone: Edinburgh 1973

3 Murray, Robin M. 'Analgesic Abuse' *British Journal of Hospital Medicine* May 1974

4 Office of Health Economics, 'The Social Content of Ill-Health' *Medicine and Society: The Changing Demands for Medical Care* London, October 1972

5 United States Department of Commerce, Social and Economic Administration *Statistical Abstract of the United States 1974: Section: Vital Statistics, Health and Nutrition*

6 Taylor, P. T. 'Some International Trends in Sickness Absence 1950–68' *British Medical Journal* 20 December 1969

7 *On the State of the Public Health, The Annual Report of the Chief Medical Officer of the Department of Health and Social Security* HMSO: London 1974

8 Quoted from Pigache, P. 'In Need of Self-Care and Control' *World Medicine* 9 April 1975

9 United States Department of Commerce, Social and Economic Administration, *Statistical Abstract of the United States 1974: Section: Vital Statistics, Health and Nutrition*

10 Roth, Sir Martin 'The Success Story of Modern Psychiatry in Britain: Part One' *The Times* 10 February 1975

11 United States Department of Commerce, Social and Economic Administration, *Statistical Abstract of the United States 1974: Section: Vital Statistics, Health and Nutrition*

12 Blyth, Jeffrey. US Report 'Hunt for killer in cancer boom' *GP* 2 January 1976

13 Gray, P. G. and others. 'Adult Dental Health in England and Wales in 1968' *British Dental Journal* Vol 129 No 3 and No 4, 4 and 18 August 1970

14 Macpherson, Lawrie *Nature Hits Back* (Second Edition) Methuen & Co Ltd: London 1936

15 Price, Weston A. *Nutrition and Physical Degeneration: A Comparison of Primitive and Modern Diets and Their Effects* Published by the author: California 1945

16 Scott-Harden, W. G. 'Radiological Investigation of Peptic Ulcer' *British Journal of Hospital Medicine* August 1973

17 'Smoking Causes 100,100 UK Deaths a Year' *Medical News – Tribune* 23 October 1970

18 'US Heart Death Rate Decreasing' *General Practitioner* 17 May 1974

19 Bedford, R. *The Deadly Cloud, A Health Educational Council Publication on Smoking and How to Give It Up* 1971

20 'Smokers' Children are Less Healthy' *GP* 22 August 1969

21 '... But in USA They Are Taking it Seriously' *Medical News* 3 November 1967

22 Camp, J. 'A Million Alcoholics' *World Medicine* 8 May 1974

23 Williams, Lincoln *Tomorrow Will be Sober* Cassell & Co Ltd: Second edition, London 1961

24 Ulrich, R. *Coffee and Caffeine* John Wright & Sons Ltd: Bristol 1958

25 Greden John F. 'Anxiety or Caffeinism: A Diagnostic Dilemma', *Am. J. Psychiatry*, 131, 10. Oct. 1974

26 Report from the Boston Collaborative Drug Surveillance Program 'Coffee Drinking and Acute Myocardial Infarction' *The Lancet*, 2, 1278, 1972

27 Misirlioghu, Y. I. 'Coffee Drinking and Acute Myocardial Infarction', letter to *The Lancet*, 1, 46, 1973

28 'Caffeine, coffee, and cancer', *British Medical Journal*, 1st May 1976

29 'Iron absorption and tea drinking', abstract in *Modern Medicine* April 1976, quoting paper by P. B. Disler and others, published in *Gut*, 16:193–200, 1975

30 Ryle, A. *Neurosis in the Ordinary Family* Tavistock Publications Ltd: London 1967

31 'International Use of Tranquilizers', leading article, *British Medical Journal* 3 August 1974

32 Conolly, J. 'Stress and Coronary Artery Disease' *British Journal of Hospital Medicine* February 1974
33 Toffler, A. *Future Shock* Pan Books Ltd: London 1970

2 The principles of natural therapy

1 For the philosophical implications of a classification according to individual parts on the one hand and the idea of the whole on the other, as evident in scientific medicine and Natural Therapy respectively, see Ledermann, E. K. *Philosophy and Medicine* Tavistock Publications Ltd: London 1970; J. B. Lippincott Co: Philadelphia 1970

3 Food and your health

1 Hall, Ross Hume. *Food for Nought: The Decline in Nutrition* Harper & Row, 1974
2 'Anti-obesity Drugs', *Mims Magazine*, Haymarket Publishing Ltd., London W.1, December 1975
3 Sedgwick, J. P. 'A Comprehensive Guide to the Problems of Simple Obesity' *GP* 10 October 1969
4 Silverstone, J. Trevor, 'Psychological and Social Aspects of Obesity' *British Journal of Hospital Medicine* July 1973
5 Ibid.
6 Cleave, T. L. and Campbell, G. D. 'Research Review: The Saccharine Disease' *Medical News* 16 June 1967
7 Cleave, T. L. and Campbell, G. D. *Diabetes, Coronary Thrombosis and the Saccharine Disease* John Wright & Sons Ltd: Bristol 1966
8 Cleave, T. L. and Campbell, G. D. 'Research Review: The Saccharine Disease' *Medical News* 16 June 1967
9 Balfour, E. B. *The Living Soil* Gives evidence of the importance to human health of soil vitality, with special reference to post-war planning, Faber & Faber Ltd: London 1943
10 Ibid.
11 Balfour, Lady Eve. 'Land Health' *Journal of the Soil Association* Vol 2 No 2 February 1974
12 Ibid.
13 See Blake, Michael. 'Only the Details are Different' *Journal of the Soil Association* Vol 1 No 9 December 1973
14 The danger arising from the use of nitrates is dealt with in Walters, Harry. *Nitrates in Soil, Plants and Animals* Leicester 1970; a pamphlet reprinted from the *Journal of the Soil Association* Vol 16

15 Shears, C. Curtis. *Nutritional Science and Health Education* published by the author, 1974

16 Ibid.

17 Ibid.

18 Ibid.

19 'Making Food Efficient' *World Medicine* 24 February 1971

20 'Substitute Foods and Safety' *The Vegetarian* November 1974

21 Shears, C. Curtis. *Nutritional Science and Health Education* published by the author, 1974

22 Davis, J. G. 'The Food Industry in AD 2000', *Journal of the Royal Society of Arts*, 1966, 114

23 Runcie, J. Hilditch, T. E. 'Energy Provision, Tissue Utilisation and Weight Loss in Prolonged Starvation' *British Medical Journal* 18 May 1974

24 Drenick, E. J. and others 'Prolonged Starvation as Treatment for Severe Obesity' *Journal of the American Medical Association* 187: 1964; summarised in *Modern Medicine of Great Britain* April 1965

25 Shelton, H. M. *Fasting Can Save Your Life* Natural Hygiene Press: Chicago 1964

26 Heun, E. 'Regeneration durch Hungern, Fasten and Rohsäfte' *Hippokrates* Heft 15, Stuttgart 1960

27 Shears, C. Curtis *Nutritional Science and Health Education* published by the author, 1974

28 Hare, D. C. 'A Therapeutic Trial of a Raw Vegetable Diet in Chronic Rheumatic Conditions' *Proceedings of the Royal Society of Medicine* Vol 30 No 1 1936

29 Hare, D. C. and Pillman-Williams, E. C. 'Vitamin C Output in Diet Treatment of Rheumatoid Arthritis' *The Lancet* Vol 1 No 20 1938

30 Carlson, L. A. and Froberg, S. O. 'Blood Liquid and Glucose Levels During a Ten-day Period of Low-Calorific Intake and Exercise in Man' *Metabolism* Vol 16 No 624 1967

31 Kuratsune, Massamori. 'Experiment on Low Nourishment with Raw Vegetables' *Kyushu Memoirs of Medical Sciences* 2 June 1951

32 Allen, R. J. L., Brook, M. and Broadbent, S. R. 'The Variability of Vitamin C in Our Diet' *British Journal of Nutrition* Vol 22 No 555 1968

33 Burrell, R. J. W., Roach, W. A. and Shadwell, A. 'Esophageal Cancer in the Bantu of the Transkel Associated with Mineral Deficiency in Garden Plants' *Journal of the National Cancer Institute* Vol 36 No 201 1966

34 Segall, J. J. 'Cardiovascular Disease and Peptic Ulcer', Letter, *British Medical Journal*, 1, 152, 1975

35 Davies, D. F. and others. 'Food antibodies and Myocardial Infarction' *The Lancet*, 1, 1012, 1974

36 Annard, J. C., 'Hypothesis: Heated Milk Protein and Thrombosis', *J. Atheroscl res.* 7, 797, 1967

37 Jacobson, B. 'Stones of Affluence', *World Medicine*, August 27. 1975

38 Crouch, T. H. 'Dietary Immunology: An Hypothesis', *New Zealand med. J.*, 372, 1972

39 Davies, D. F. and others. 'Food Antibodies and Myocardial Infarction' *The Lancet*, 1, 1012, 1974

40 Cleave, T. L. and Campbell, G. D., *Diabetes, Coronary Thrombosis and the Saccharine Disease*, John Wright & Sons Ltd. Bristol 1966

41 Shears, C. Curtis, *Nutritional Science and Health Education*, publ. by the author 1974

42 Ibid.

43 Selling, Lowell S. and Ferraro, Mary Anna, *The Psychology of Diet and Nutrition*, John Lane, The Bodley Head Ltd., London 1947

44 Silverstone, J. Trevor, 'Psychological and Social Aspects of Obesity', *British Journal of Hospital Medicine*, July 1973

45 'Cancer death rate rise puzzles doctors', US Report in *GP*, 28 November, 1975

46 'Bad diet may pave the way to cancer', US Report in *GP*, 19 December 1975

4 Health and your bowel

1 Hawley, P. R. 'Carcinoma of the Colon' *British Journal of Hospital Medicine* February 1974

2 Eastwood, M. A. and Mitchell, W. D. 'The Place of Vegetable Fibre in Diet' *British Journal of Hospital Medicine* January 1974

3 Cleave, T. L. and Campbell, G. D. *Diabetes, Coronary Thrombosis and the Saccharine Disease* John Wright & Sons Ltd: Bristol 1966

4 La Rue, A. 'Effects of Acidified Milk on Intestinal Pathogens' *Canadian Medical Association Journal* Vol 83 No 1002 1960

5 Raffle, E. J. 'Yoghurt in Gastro-Enteritis of Infancy' letter to *The Lancet* Vol 2 No 1106 1956

6 Ferrer, F. P. and Boyd, L. J. 'Effect of Yoghurt with Prune-whip on Constipation' *American Journal Dig. Dis* Vol 22 1955

7 Ask-Upmark, E. 'A New Remedy for Migraine' letter to *The Lancet* Vol 2 No 446 1966

8 Quoted from Wittkower, E. D. *Einfluss der Gemütsbewegungen auf den Körper* (Second Edition) Sensen Verlag: Vienna and Leipzig 1937

9 Shelton, H. M. *Fasting Can Save Your Life* Natural Hygiene Press: Chicago 1964

5 The breath of life

1 Jones, N. L. and Fletcher, C. M. 'The Management of Chronic Bronchitis and Emphysema' *Hospital Medicine* December 1967

2 Blyth, J. 'Take a Deep Breath. . . .' US Report *GP* 27 September 1974

3 'Authorities "Totally Ignorant" of Pollution Hazards' *GP* 5 May 1972

6 Natural stimulation and your skin

1 St. John Lyburn, E. F. 'Nine Clinical Achievements of Therapeutic Sweating' *Hospital Times* 6 October 1970

2 Müller-Limmroth, W. and Ruffman, A. 'Experimentelle Untersuchungen über die physiologischen Sauna-Wirkungen auf den gesunden Menschen' *Hippokrates* Heft 23 Stuttgart 15 December 1962

3 Krauss, H. 'Physikalisch-diätetische Therapie der entzündlichen Rheumakrankheiten' *Hippokrates* Heft 5 Stuttgart 1961

4. 'Sauna Baths Prove to be Harmful' *Medical News-Tribune* Vol 2 No 43 23 October 1970

5 Hoff, A. 'Allgemeines und Spezielles aus der Naturheilkunde' *Hippokrates* Stuttgart 31 August 1947

6 Kneipp, Father. *My Water Cure* William Blackwood & Sons Ltd: Edinburgh 1891

7 Franke, K. 'Die Bedeutung der kleinen Hydrotherapie (nach Kneipp) für die Prävention und Rehabilitation von Arthritis und Kollagen-Krankheiten am, Gefäszsystem' *Hippokrates* Heft 3 Stuttgart 1961

8 Velse, F. 'Physikalische und diätetische Behandlung des Bluthochdrucks' *Archiv für Physikalische Therapie* Heft 4 1966

9 For a summary of the effects of the ground and the air on the skin see Kunze, Gerhard. *Physiatrie, Naturärztliche Rundschau* January, August 1932

10 'Sun, Wind and the Skin' *British Medical Journal* 13 July 1974

11 Rollier, A. *Heliotheraphy* Oxford Medical Publications: London; Henry Frowde and Hodder & Stoughton Ltd: London 1923

12 Ibid.

13 Rollier, A. *The International Factory Clinic for the Treatment by Sun and Work of Indigent Cases of 'Surgical' Tuberculosis* Librarie Payot et Cie: Paris 1929

14 Mayer, Edward. *Radiation and Climatic Therapy of Chronic Pulmonary Diseases with Special Reference to Natural and Artificial Heliotherapy, X-Ray and Climatic Therapy of Chronic Pulmonary Diseases and All Forms of Tuberculosis* The Williams & Wilkins Company: Baltimore 1944

7 Posture, exercise and relaxation
1 Neill, Charles A. *Poise and Relaxation* A Family Doctor Publication: London (now O/P)
2 Ibid.
3 Crutchfield, Kenneth. 'Exercise' in Cooper Ernest (ed) *Health in the Home: The Food Reform and Nature Cure Manual* The London Health Centre Ltd. and the National Association of Health Stores: London 1948
4 Cooper, Kenneth H. *The New Aerobics* Bantam Books Ltd: New York, USA 1970
5 Ibid.
6 Semple, Thomas. 'Exercise in Prevention of Coronary Heart Disease' *Health Magazine* Vol 2 No. 1 Spring 1974
7 Houston, J. C., Joiner, C. L. and Trounce, J. R. *A Short Textbook of Medicine* English Universities Press Ltd: London 1968
8 Lübken, W. 'Bewegung und Hydrotherapie in der Diabetesbehandlung' *Hippokrates* Heft 8 Stuttgart 1961
9 Schultz, Johannes H. and Luthe, Wolfgang. *Autogenic Training, a Psychophysiologic Approach in Psychotherapy* Grune & Stratton Inc: New York 1959

8 Allies to Natural Therapy
1 See Ledermann, E. K. 'Homoeopathy and Natural Therapeutics' *The British Homoeopathic Journal* Vol XXXV No 1 May 1945
2 See Ledermann, E. K. 'The Philosophical and Scientific Basis of Alopathic and Homoeopathic Medicine' *The British Homoeopathic Journal* Vol XXXIV Nos 2, 3 September 1944
3 See Ledermann, E. K. 'Implications of Hahnemannian Homoeopathy' *The British Homoeopathic Journal* Vol XLVI No 4 October 1957
4 See for example the animal experiments which demonstrate such connections, quoted in Mann, Felix. *Acupuncture: The Ancient Chinese Art of Healing* William Heinemann Medical Books Ltd: London 1971

5 See for instance Moss, Louis. *Acupuncture and You* Paul Elek Books Ltd: London 1972

6 See for instance Stiefvater, Eric H. *What is Acupuncture? How does it Work?* (Second Edition) Health Science Press: 1971

7 Renard, Paul. 'Pathologie-Psychologie et Acupuncture' (Second instalment) *Revue Trimestrielle de l'Organisation pour l'Étude et le Développement de l'Acupuncture* 11e année No 41 July, August, September 1974

8 Bergsmann, Otto. *Objektivierung der Akupunktur als Problem der Regulationsphysiologie* Verlag Haug: Heidelberg 1974

9 Hoag, Marshall, Cole, Wilbur V. and Bradford, Spencer G. *Osteopathic Medicine* The Blakiston Division/McGraw-Hill Inc: New York 1969

10 Ibid.

11 Bradbury, Parnell *The Mechanics of Healing* Peter Owen Ltd: London 1967

12 Dicke, Elisabeth, *Meine Bindegewebsmassage*, Hippokrates-Verlag, 2. edition 1954
English version: Ebner, Maria, *Connective Tissue Massage, Theory and Therapeutic Application*, E. & S. Livingstone, Edinburgh & London 1962

Index

acid-forming foods 40
acne vulgaris (case history)
  130–2
acupuncture 111–13
aerobics 102–3, 122
affusions 79
air pollution 67–9
air treatment 80–2
  bath 81–2
alcoholism 10
Alexander, Matthias 86
alkaline-producing foods 40
amorphous carbon 110
anaemia, pernicious 4, 84
anemone-pulsatilla 108
angina pectoris 36, 75
anorexia nervosa 22, 56
antibiotics 4, 21, 30
appendicitis 22
appendix 26
appetite 57
  'appestat' 25
arthritis, osteo 40
  case history 123
  rheumatoid 6, 39, 40, 74
  case history 126–8
aspirin 5
asthma 39, 115
  and cigarette smoking 9
autogenic training 103–6
avocado pears 54

bacillus proteus 127
bacteria 28
baths 79
Bergsmann, Dr Otto 113
Bischko, Dr J. 113
blood pressure, high 80
boils (case history) 120–1

bowel flora 26, 62
Bradbury, Parnell 115
bran 49, 61
bread 31
breathing 70
bronchitis 20, 39, 82
  and cigarette smoking 9

caffeine 11–13
calcium 46
calories 23, 24, 41
cancer 6, 29, 30, 48, 59, 61
  and caffeine 13
  of the large bowel 60, 61
  lung 4
    and cigarette smoking 9, 10
  of the stomach 8
carbohydrates 23ff., 42
carbon monoxide 67, 68, 73
catarrh (case history) 125–6
chiropractic 115
cholesterol 52, 72
  serum 62
cigarette smoking 9, 10
cinchona 122
cold treatment 75–82
  water 75–80
  air 80–2
colic 61, 75
colitis (case history) 121–3
colonic-irrigation 64–5
compress, cold water 77–9
constipation 8, 62, 63, 65, 117
conventional medicine 3, 4, 27,
  107
Cooper, Dr Kenneth M. 102
copper 48
coronary disease 26
cramp 118

Crutchfield, Kenneth 92
customs of eating 58

dental caries 7
dermatitis 35, 63
  and caffeine 11
diabetes 4, 26, 103
diarrhoea 21, 35, 62, 65
  and caffeine 12
  during fast 38
Dicke, Mrs Elisabeth 116
diet
  full 41
  grape 35, 125
  milk 34
  raw fruit and vegetable 39, 40,
    41
  Schrott 33–4
  simple balanced 48
digitalis 4
diverticulitis 61
drug picture 108–10
dyspepsia 8

eczema, and caffeine 11
eggs 52
emphysema, and cigarette
  smoking 9
enema 64
enzymes 31, 39
exercises
  against constipation 63, 64
  lying 98–100
  on hands and knees 101
  standing 92–8, 101

fasting 35–9
fats 23, 42
  polyunsaturated 42

fluorine 69
froment 49

gall bladder 26, 115
Ghenanda Sambita 63, 64
glaucoma, and caffeine 11
gout 36
growth hormones 30

haemorrhoids 26
Hahnemann, Dr Samuel 109
heart disease 9, 85, 102
  (see also coronary disease)
  ischaemic 6, 14
  and cigarette smoking 8
heart failure 4
  case history 128–9
heat treatment 72
  dry 73
  local application 73
  moist 72
hepatic cirrhosis 10
herbicides 59
homoeopathy 107–11
honey 52
humus 28
hunger 56
hydrotherapy, combinations in
  79–80

iatrogenic disease 5
immunization 4
inflammation
  of appendix 26
  of gall bladder 26
  of kidneys 26, 39, 115
  case history 129–30
insulin 4
iron 46

kali arsenicosum 129
  bromatum 131
  iodatum 130
kidneys 4, 26, 34, 35, 47, 73, 115
  and caffeine 12, 13
Kneipp, Father 77

lachesis 109
lactobacilli 62, 63
laxatives 64
lead 69
liver 112
  cirrhosis of (case history)
    124–5
lungs 67–70

magnesium 46
massage 116
  professional 116
  self- 116–19
measles 39
mental illness 6, 22
mental stress 13–15
metabolism
  basal 11
  fat (and fibre content) 62
milk 32, 50–2
  diet 34
mineral salts 23, 46–7
molybdenum 48
myocardial infarction
  and milk 51
  and caffeine 13

natrium muriaticum (common
    salt) 108
natural stimuli 19, 20
nausea, and caffeine 12
Neill, Charles A. 86

nephritis (case history) 129–30
neuritis 10
neurosis 13
nitrates 29
nux vomica 133

obesity 23, 24, 56
oedema 35
organic farming 28
osteopathic lesion 114
osteopathy 113–15
oxalate 51

paracetamol 5
peritonitis 85
perspiration (sweating) 72–4,
    76, 78, 80
pesticides 29, 59
phenacitin 5
phlebitis 78, 80
posture 86–92
potassium 36, 47, 74
Priessnitz, Vinzenz 76
proteins 23, 26, 32, 42
psychodietetics 55–9
pyelitis 27
pyrogen 122

Renard, Dr Paul 113
rice 52
Rollier, A. 83–5

saccharine disease 25–7
sauna bath 73–4
schizophrenia 6
Schultz, J. H. 104
sclerosis
  arterio 20, 72
  and caffeine 11

sclerosis *continued*
  multiple (case history) 132–3
seeds
  pumpkin 54
  sesame 54
  sunflower 54
'silica 30' 126
sinusitis, acute (case history)
    133–4
sitting (correct posture) 91
skin 71, 119
  irritation 4
  virus infection (case history)
    121–3
sodium chloride 34, 47, 74
soya beans 52
spine 86–8
spinology 115
sprouting grains 53, 132
standing (correct posture) 88–90
starvation 36, 37
sulphur dioxide 68
sun treatment 82–5
suppository 64
swathing (wet) 79

symbolization 58

tannins 13
thalidomide 5
thyroid gland 4
tonsillitis 39, 78
tonsils, and self-massage 118
trace elements 23, 48
tuberculosis 20, 83, 85

ulcers 8, 14, 26, 39, 50, 63, 115
  varicose (case history) 124

varicose veins 26
vitamins 4, 23, 31, 40, 43–6, 49,
    84
  description and sources of
    supply 43–6
vomiting (during fast) 38
  and caffeine 12

walking, correct posture 91–2
water cure 77

zinc 48